Real-time Ultrasound in Obstetrics

To Jane

Real-time Ultrasound in Obstetrics

EDITED BY

M. J. Bennett

MD MRCOG FCOG(SA)
Senior Lecturer and Consultant
Institute of Obstetrics and Gynaecology
Queen Charlotte's Hospital for Women
London

AND

S. Campbell

MB BS FRCOG
Professor of Obstetrics and Gynaecology
King's College Hospital Medical School
London

Blackwell Scientific Publications
OXFORD LONDON EDINBURGH
BOSTON MELBOURNE

© 1980 by
Blackwell Scientific Publications
Editorial offices:
Osney Mead, Oxford OX2 0EL
8 John Street, London WC1N 2ES
9 Forrest Road, Edinburgh EH1 2QH
214 Berkeley Street, Carlton
    Victoria 3053, Australia

First published 1980

Printed and bound in Great Britain by
Butler & Tanner Ltd
Frome and London

DISTRIBUTORS

USA
    Blackwell Mosby Book Distributors
    11830 Westline Industrial
    St Louis, Missouri 63141

Canada
    Blackwell Mosby Book Distributors
    86 Northline Road, Toronto
    Ontario, M4B 3E5

Australia
    Blackwell Scientific Book
    Distributors
    214 Berkeley Street, Carlton
    Victoria 3053

British Library
Cataloguing in Publication Data

Real-time ultrasound in obstetrics.
    1. Diagnosis, Ultrasonic   2. Obstetrics –
    Diagnosis
    I. Bennett, M J   II. Campbell, S
    618.2'2   RG527.5.U48

ISBN 0–632–00585–8

Contents

Contributors

A. H. Adam MB ChB MRCOG
Diagnostic Ultrasound Unit, Department of Midwifery, Queen Mother's
Hospital, Glasgow

M. J. Bennett MD MRCOG FCOG(SA)
Senior Lecturer and Consultant, Institute of Obstetrics and Gynaecology,
Queen Charlotte's Hospital for Women, London

R. J. Blackwell BSc MSc MInstP CEng MIEE
Principal Physicist, Department of Medical Physics & Bio-Engineering,
University College Hospital, London

Stuart Campbell MB BS FRCOG
Professor of Obstetrics and Gynaecology, King's College Hospital Medical
School, London

D. Cooper MSc PhD
Senior Programmer and Analyst, King's College Hospital Medical School,
London

Greggory R. Devore MD
Department of Obstetrics and Gynecology, Yale University School of Medicine, New Haven, Connecticut

Gerhard Gennser MD
Consultant Obstetrician and Gynaecologist, University Hospital, Malmö,
Sweden

John C. Hobbins MD
Professor of Perinatal Medicine, Yale University School of Medicine, New
Haven, Connecticut

P. J. Lewis MD PhD MRCP
Senior Lecturer in Clinical Pharmacology and Honorary Consultant Physician, Royal Postgraduate Medical School, Hammersmith, London

D. J. Little MB BS MRCOG
Research Registrar in Obstetrics and Gynaecology, King's College Hospital Medical School, London

Hylton B. Meire MB BS LRCP MRCS DMRD DObsRCOG FRCR
Consultant in Ultrasound and Consultant Radiologist, Clinical Research Centre, Division of Radiology, Harrow, Middlesex

Elena Olivier
Clinical Pharmacology Unit, Institute of Obstetrics and Gynaecology, Queen Charlotte's Hospital for Women, London

A. B. Roberts MB ChB MRCOG
Research Registrar in Obstetrics and Gynaecology, King's College Hospital Medical School, London

H. P. Robinson MB ChB MRCOG
Diagnostic Ultrasound Unit, Department of Midwifery, Queen Mother's Hospital, Glasgow

W. Vletter
Department of Cardiovascular Research, Erasmus University, Rotterdam

R. Vosters MD
Senior Registrar in Obstetrics and Gynaecology, Erasmus University, Rotterdam

J. W. Wladimiroff MD PhD
Reader in Obstetrics and Gynaecology, Erasmus University, Rotterdam

Preface

The rapid development of real-time ultrasonic equipment in recent years has been paralleled by the acceptance by obstetricians of the vital role this equipment plays in clinical obstetric practice. Not only does today's obstetrician rely upon ultrasound for the determination of gestational age, placental position and the presence of multiple gestation, but more and more is he relying upon the ultrasonic assessment of intra-uterine growth. The potential for obtaining information about fetal development and dynamic functions is now only beginning to be utilized.

This book incorporates a balance between the use to which this equipment can be put in ordinary obstetric practice and the areas of investigation which will contribute to a better understanding of fetal functions in the future. The authors are all experts in their own fields and have been chosen for this reason.

We hope that this book will be of assistance both to obstetricians involved primarily in clinical practice and to those wishing to advance the frontiers of knowledge in fetal medicine.

Michael Bennett   *April 1980*
Stuart Campbell

CHAPTER 1

The basic physical principles of real-time ultrasound scanning

R. J. Blackwell

The physical principles of real-time ultrasound scanning are much the same as those involved in conventional ultrasound scanning. However, there are certain important differences. Real-time ultrasound scanning frequently uses an array of transducer elements employed in a number of different combinations and producing distinctive sound field patterns. The clarity of a real-time scan is not simply a function of the resolution, which can be described in physical terms, but is influenced by the ability of the eye to perceive moving structures more clearly than stationary ones. One of the most significant differences of real-time scanners, at the present, is the fact that the scanning instrument is relatively 'user transparent'. That is to say, the operator does not have to be highly skilled to operate the equipment but may concentrate on the interpretation of the results. Because of this, the emphasis of any physical foundation must shift from a detailed understanding of the equipment and controls towards a grasp of the physical principles involved in the interpretation of the scan. In particular, an understanding of the principal types of artefact must be obtained.

We shall commence by examining, in general terms, how a real-time picture is derived, and then go on to consider some of the major artefacts occurring in the scan, and finally mention the techniques used in some of the more recent types of real-time scanner.

THE REAL-TIME SCAN

Fig. 1.1 shows a typical real-time scan of a fetal head. The picture consists of white dots, representing echoes, on a black background. The echo pattern represents a cross-section of the tissues immediately underneath the probe. The section is that which would be seen if the probe were used as a cleaver to cut through the body. It must always be remembered that only a thin section of tissues is viewed in any one picture and that the probe must be moved around to give a three-dimensional impression of the tissue structures.

1

Three distinct areas have been identified on the scan. One (labelled A) is completely devoid of echoes. Such black regions are called anechoic and frequently relate to fluid regions, such as the amniotic fluid (arrowed). They may, alternatively, be solid but acoustically homogeneous, such as much of the fetal brain tissue. In this case, the echoes are so small that their amplitude falls below the detection threshold of the equipment. The second area exhibits a clear white outline (S); echoes of this type are generated by strong reflectors such as the fetal skull. The third area (G) has a grey, mottled appearance, and is generated by small echoes arising from tissue infra-structure, in this case, the structure of an anterior placenta. The size, or amplitude, of each echo is represented on the scan as a shade of grey, the darker shades arising from weaker echoes. These grey scale-echoes give an impression of 'tissue texture'.

If we were to 'zoom' into the part of the picture showing the fetal head we would obtain a scan such as that shown in Fig. 1.2. The picture is clearly composed of a number of faint, parallel straight lines, called the timebase lines, which are made momentarily bright each time an echo is received by the equipment

The way in which these lines are displayed is shown in Fig. 1.3. The probe, which is placed on the patient's abdomen, is composed of a series of trans-

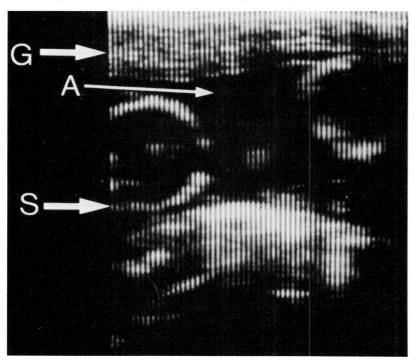

Fig. 1.1 An ultrasonic scan is made up of anechoic areas A, white outlines from specular echoes S, and grey areas G, indicating tissue texture, arising from scattered echoes.

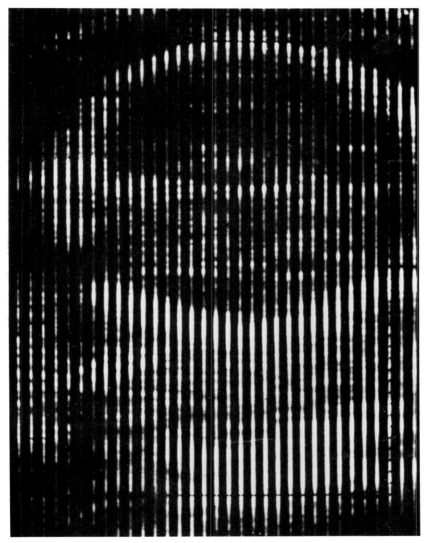

Fig. 1.2 Real-time scan of a fetal head. The parallel timebase lines are increased in brightness each time an echo is received.

ducer elements packed together in a straight line to form a linear array. (A transducer is a device which transforms energy from one form to another, in this case a voltage pulse into a pulse of ultrasound or vice versa.) The first element in the array is selected by an electronic switch. A pulse of ultrasound is generated and the echoes are received by the element. At the same moment that the pulse of sound is generated, the timebase starts to move across the screen of the display oscilloscope parallel to the left-hand edge. When the timebase has reached the end of its travel the spot is returned to

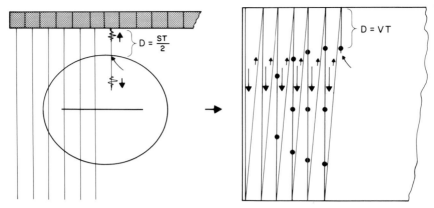

Fig. 1.3 There is a direct correspondence between the physical situation (left) and the display (right). The spacing of the timebase lines is determined by the distance between the transducer elements in the array, and the timebase speed V corresponds to the average speed of sound in tissue S. The depth D, from which an echo originates, is derived from the time T required for a pulse of sound to travel from the probe to the reflector and back again.

the top of the screen and moved across by a distance corresponding to the spacing of the elements in the array. The cycle is now repeated by the second element in the array and the timebase again moves across the screen parallel to the first timebase line. The process is continued sequentially along the array to form a scan frame. Each frame is completed in less than $\frac{1}{40}$ sec. and so moving structures can be visualized.

The position of any echo in the display is determined from the time which elapses between the pulse of sound being generated and the echo being received. Using the relationship that distance is the product of speed multiplied by time, we can calculate the position of an echo-producing structure, relative to the probe, from the time delay, providing we are prepared to assume a speed of sound in tissue. Unfortunately, in practice, sound has different speeds in different tissues — the variation between different soft tissues·being about 4%. This limits the accuracy of the technique. Of course, the sound pulse has to travel out to the anatomical structure and back again to the probe, so the distance between the probe and the structure is the product of the assumed speed multiplied by the elapsed time, divided by two. In order to position the echo correctly on the oscilloscope timebase, the velocity of the timebase across the screen must be equal to the speed of sound in tissues divided by two if a full-sized picture is to be obtained, or scaled appropriately if a full-sized picture is not desired.

It will be clear that, in order to position a spot accurately, we must know not only the distance between the probe and the structure but the direction in which the structure lies. This is made possible by generating pencil beams of ultrasound. Ultrasound, rather than audible sound, is used in order to generate these beams, and the required frequencies are about a hundred times the audible limit, i.e. 2 MHz (the Hertz is the SI unit of frequency, one Hertz being one event per second). In addition to producing well defined, narrow beams of sound, very short pulses of sound may be produced at these frequencies. This enables very accurate timing to be performed and makes it possible to discriminate between echoes arising from closely spaced structures.

WHY WAVELENGTH MATTERS

In Fig. 1.4 we see a representation of an ultrasound beam. The transducer, at the left, is made of piezoelectric (more correctly ferroelectric) material

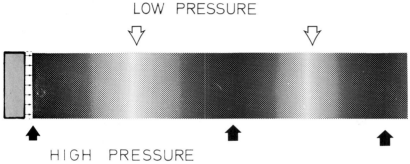

Fig. 1.4   The ultrasound beam.

which changes its dimensions in response to an electric voltage placed across its faces. The voltage has caused the front face of the transducer to move forward very rapidly and compress the tissues, resulting in a local high pressure region. This high pressure region propagates into the tissues at the speed of sound and the resultant oscillation of the molecular structure of the tissues gives rise to a series of high pressure regions interspersed by low pressure regions moving through the tissues. Such pressure fluctuations are called longitudinal compression waves. The distance between pressure peaks is called the wavelength (symbol λ) and the rate at which pressure peaks are received at one point in the tissue is called the frequency.

The speed of the ultrasonic soundwave is determined by the density and elasticity of the tissue structure. Any change in either factor, such as occurs at a tissue boundary, results in a small proportion of the sound energy (typically about 0.5%) being reflected back towards the transducer (Fig. 1.5). If the tissue boundary is flat and large compared to the wavelength, then 'mirrorlike' or specular reflection occurs. If, however, the reflecting structure is small compared to the wavelength, then sound is scattered, or re-radiated, in all directions from the reflector. Specular reflection is relatively strong, and gives rise to the white outlines in the scan. Scattered reflection, on the other hand, is very weak, but is responsible for the bulk of the echoes in

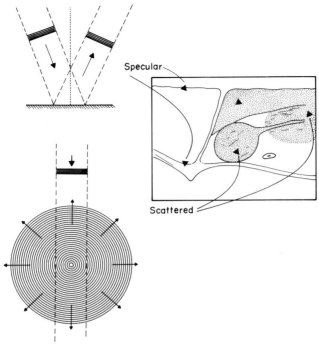

Fig. 1.5   Sound is reflected from large smooth surfaces in a mirrorlike or 'specular' fashion. Specular reflection is responsible for many of the strong white outlines on the scan. Small discontinuities within tissue masses give rise to small omnidirectional echoes known as 'scatter'. The grey tones on the scan relate to the amount of scatter received and give an impression of tissue 'texture'.

the picture and also fulfils the important role of indicating small changes in tissue texture. This is useful, for instance, in differentiating between placenta and lower uterine segment. Specular reflection is strongly dependent upon the angle of incidence of the sound beam to the surface, and a slight deviation from normal causes the sound pulse to be reflected away from the transducer so that virtually no echo energy is received by the probe. On the other hand, scattered reflection is almost independent of angle, and the sound energy, although very weak, always returns to the probe. The amount of sound scattered back towards the transducer is dependent upon the relative size of the scattering object and the sound wavelength. If the wavelength is halved then the amount of scatter increases approximately sixteen-fold, i.e. according to a fourth-power law. Many structures in the body are neither large and flat, nor very tiny, and in consequence an intermediate type of reflection occurs.

Fig. 1.6 shows the way in which a sound beam spreads out as the size or aperture of the transducer is reduced. The sound beam from a small transducer remains parallel for only a limited distance from the probe and then starts to diverge. The parallel section is known as the near field or Fresnel

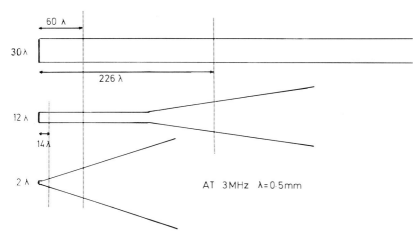

Fig. 1.6 The funnel-shaped ultrasound field diverges more rapidly as the face of the transducer is reduced in size. Thus, it is advantageous to use a transducer of width 2λ rather than 30λ if all the structures of interest lie within 60λ of the probe face. If structures 'deep' in the body are to be imaged a relatively wide (about 10 mm) transducer is required.

Zone, and the divergent section as the far field or Fraunhoffer Zone. The beam is thus funnel-shaped, with the angle of divergence decreasing as the size of the transducer is increased. A large transducer gives a well defined parallel-sided beam right throughout the body, but the beam is broadened by an unacceptable amount. In contrast, a medium-sized transducer gives a narrow beam near the transducer, enabling greater precision in locating an echo, whereas the beam width in the divergent section exceeds that of the large transducer for only the most distal structures. Thus, in selecting the size of the transducer, a compromise has to be made between obtaining a narrow, well-defined beam near the probe, and accepting the limitations resulting from a broad beam, with imprecise location of echoes, for distal structures. In general, real-time instruments are designed to have a probe width of about 16 wavelengths, i.e. 8 mm at a frequency of 3 MHz. It is clear that, if an array consists of 64 transducer elements, each one of them 8 mm in length, then the probe length would exceed 50 cm. This situation would be quite unacceptable and so refined techniques must be used.

If, to produce the first pulse, the first 4 elements in the array are triggered together, then a sound pulse is produced as if it had come from a transducer with an aperture equivalent to 4 element widths, thus achieving reasonable beam characteristics (Fig. 1.7). To produce the second pulse we do not use the next 4 elements in the sequence, but trigger the second to fifth elements together so that the beam axis moves by just 1 element width. By repeating this process 61 'effective transducers' can be produced from the 64 elements in the array. In this way, 61 pulses can be produced with a movement of

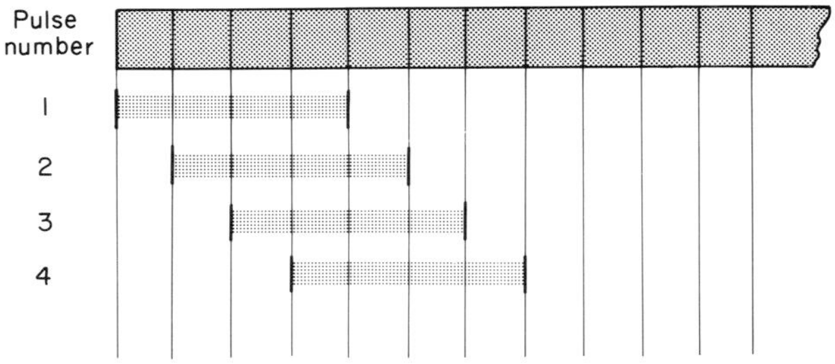

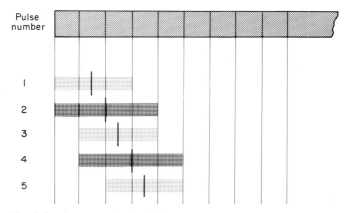

Fig. 1.7 In order to obtain a beam with narrow divergence a wide transducer must be used, but the beam must shift a short way between pulses if the scan is to contain enough lines of information for good resolution. These requirements are satisfied by using a number of small transducer elements simultaneously to generate the beam. The beam is shifted along the linear array probe by one element width by incorporating an extra element at one end of the group and making the element at the other end inactive.

the beam axis of, say, 1.5 mm between pulses, to generate a scan with a field width of 10 cm.

One problem with simple linear array scans is the 'zoo' effect. That is, the scan appears as if the structures in the body were viewed through a cage. In order to reduce this effect, more lines of information must be provided, and there are a number of ways in which this may be done. Ideally, the extra lines should contain extra information. One commonly used technique is to employ the system shown in Fig. 1.8. The first pulse is produced in the way already described, using the first few elements in the array as a single trans-ducer. In this technique, however, the second pulse is produced by including an extra element in the effective transducer, which thus moves the beam axis by half an element width. Thus, every other pulse follows the pattern we have already described, and intermediate pulses use an extra element shifting the beam along by an extra half element width. Further 'filling in' of detail

Fig. 1.8 A system for doubling the number of lines in the scan.

can be achieved by moving the display timebase lines a small amount on alternate frames, the intensity of each echo being interpolated from adjacent lines. Since 40 frames may be taken every second this technique does not produce any noticeable jitter on the picture and the effect is visually pleasing (Fig. 1.9).

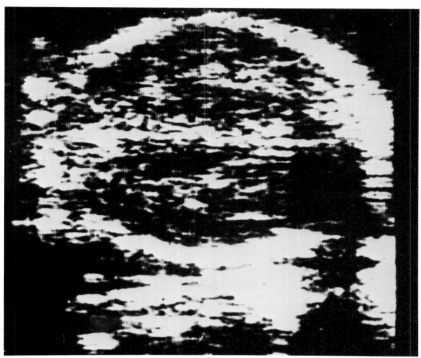

Fig. 1.9 The 'zoo effect' can almost be eliminated to give a visually pleasing effect by further increasing the number of lines. This scan of a fetal head was taken using a 'Unirad Corporation' scanner. Two extra lines of information are displayed between each pair of ultrasonically generated lines. The intensity at each point along the extra lines is obtained by linear interpolation from the intensities along the lines of the echo information.

A reduced wavelength improves the beam characteristics. Why then should we not increase the frequency of the transducer and produce very narrow pencil beams of sound? The problem is that the body attenuates sound in a directly proportional relationship to its frequency. Doubling the frequency doubles the attenuation, which in turn halves the effective penetration of the beam. A compromise has to be made by using the highest frequency which will allow the desired penetration of the beam. Ten years ago, it would have been difficult to use a frequency above 1.5 MHz. During recent years, however, 2.5 MHz and recently even 5 MHz have been employed. The ability to raise the frequency has been related to improvements in electronic technology enabling more sensitive equipment to be produced.

Reducing ultrasonic wavelength (raising frequency)	
ADVANTAGES	DISADVANTAGES
Resolution improved (directivity and pulse length)	Penetration reduced
Scattered echoes enhanced	

Fig. 1.10

We may summarize then (Fig. 1.10) by saying, use the highest frequency consistent with the desired penetration because this will improve resolution and grey scale characteristics.

ARTEFACTS

'Chinese Hat'

Fig. 1.11 shows a scan of a fetal head, but below the head is an echo (arrowed) which appears to come from a further fetal head, but which cannot be related to any obvious anatomical structure. This type of appearance is frequently seen and has been termed a 'Chinese hat' artefact, because of its shape. The origin of this type of artefact is not immediately obvious but the limited lateral resolution of the equipment is thought to be involved. In Fig. 1.12 the most sensitive part of the beam is along its axis, where the sound intensity is highest. Small, scattered echoes, arising from the central region of the beam, produce sufficiently strong echoes to be registered by the equipment. However, if these scatterers are positioned in the outer part of the beam, their echoes fall below the display threshold of the equipment and are not registered. Thus, for weak reflectors, the resolution is good because echoes are registered only when the structure is on the axis of the beam. Stronger reflectors, however, can be placed off the axis of the beam and still produce a sufficiently strong echo to register on the display. A strong reflector placed at the edge of the beam will give rise to an echo which is registered as if it had originated on the beam axis and is misregistered by quite a long way, perhaps several centimetres in error. It is for this reason that the lateral resolution of strong reflectors for most ultrasonic systems is rather poor.

However, the anticipated beam characteristics in real-time equipment are not sufficiently poor to produce the 'Chinese hat'. This type of artefact is related to the fact that the 'effective' transducer is made up of a number of smaller transducer elements. The situation is analogous to that which is experienced in optics when a beam of light is directed at a grating consisting of alternate transparent and opaque strips. It will be recalled that the main beam passes through the grating, but that diffraction effects cause side lobes which are directed at an angle to the axis of the beam. The use of a number

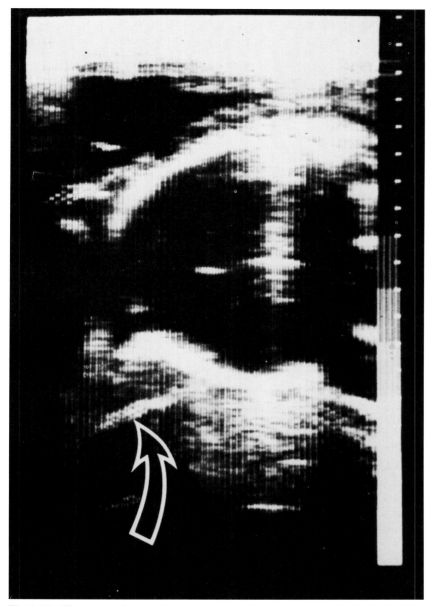

Fig. 1.11   The arrowed curve does not correspond to any structure in the body. Similar 'Chinese hat' artefacts are generated when strongly reflective areas are present in the scan.

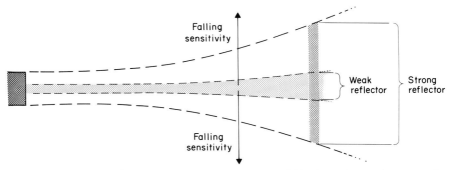

Fig. 1.12 Diagram illustrating how effective beam width depends on the type of reflector. A strong reflector may be detected over a broader area than a weak one.

of discrete transducer elements in the acoustic case similarly causes diffraction effects so that grating lobes make the beam rather wide (Fig. 1.13).

A very strong reflector, such as the distal wall of the fetal skull, may register an echo from the side lobe, even when the main beam is at a considerable

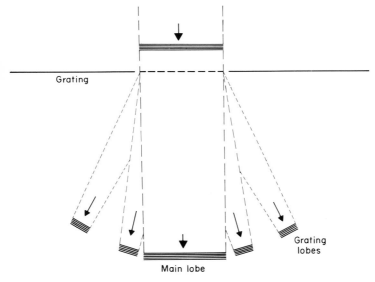

Fig. 1.13 The beam produced by a linear array has quite strong side lobes. The transducer elements are analogous to the transparent regions in an optical grating. The effect is to increase the beam divergence.

distance from the reflector. The geometry of the situation causes the echo to be displayed on the beam axis at an equivalent distance to that between the reflector and the transducer (Fig. 1.14). Fig. 1.15 shows how this distance increases as the beam is stepped across the array, causing the artefactual echo to move progressively away from the probe in a downward arc. The problem is minimised by focussing the beam.

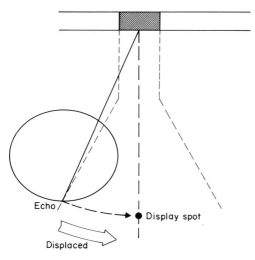

Fig. 1.14 The strong echo generated from the far side of the fetal skull is still detected when the beam axis has moved on beyond this region. The echo is registered as an artefact on the axis at a distance equal to that between the skull and the transducer.

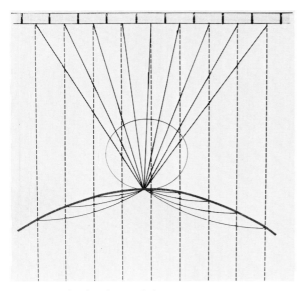

Fig. 1.15 As the ultrasonic beam moves across a strong reflector an artefactual curve is generated because the oblique distance to the transducer group increases as the beam moves away from the reflector.

Shadowing

The scan, shown in Fig. 1.16, again shows a fetal head. Below the head is the placenta. At each side of the head, shadows are cast which affect all the

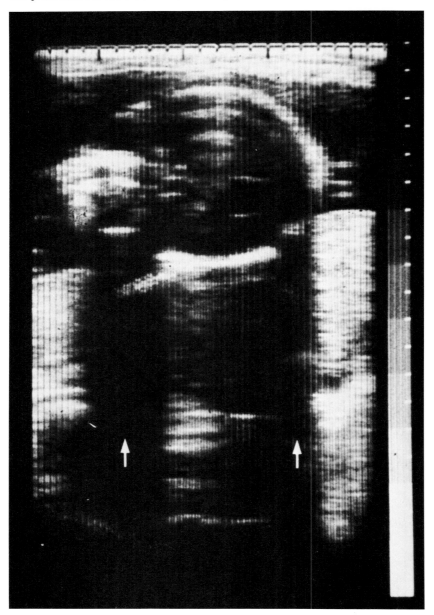

Fig. 1.16 Acoustic shadows (arrowed) occur distal to the oblique edges of strong reflectors.

distal echoes. The obvious reason for these shadows is that the skull thickness which must be traversed by the ultrasonic beam is increased because of the angle of obliquity. The attenuation coefficient of skull bone is high relative to soft tissue, resulting in a loss of beam intensity which increases with the path length through the bone. However, such shadows are also seen in soft tissue masses, for instance distal to the edge of the gall bladder, and there is an additional reason why they occur. The amount of sound reflected by a specular reflector increases with the angle of incidence. Thus, the fetal skull, instead of reflecting perhaps 1% or 2% of the incident sound, may reflect 60% or 70% (Fig. 1.17), leaving only a fraction of the original energy to pass

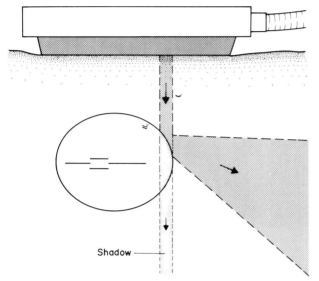

Shadow

Fig. 1.17 The quantity of sound energy reflected by a specular reflector increases markedly as the angle of incidence increases. The transmitted sound which is available for generating further echoes is correspondingly reduced. The loss of intensity results in a region of shadow.

through the head and produce echoes from distal structures. The angle between the beam and the edge of the skull causes the sound to be reflected away from the probe and it plays no part in formation of the scan.

Reverberation

Reverberation is a frequently encountered artefact affecting all scans. In its most pronounced form (Fig. 1.18) it appears as a series of linear echoes decreasing in amplitude and length. In this form it is easily recognized and ignored by the clinician. Reverberation occurs because the material of the probe is constructed from plastics and man-made ceramics which, relative to tissues, have high elastic constants. Because of this, any echo returning

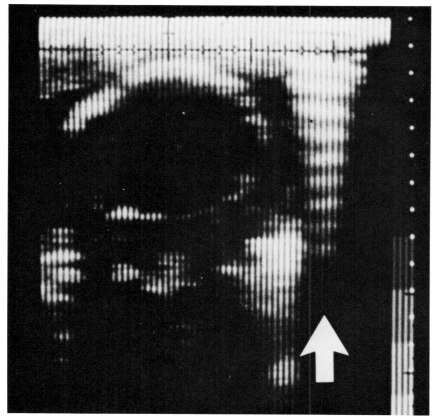

Fig. 1.18 Reverberant echoes. These are produced in this case between the probe and uterine wall. Notice that they decrease in intensity and are spaced at regular intervals.

to the probe is not completely absorbed by the transducer, but is re-reflected back down into the tissues according to the normal laws of reflection (Fig. 1.19). The energy — reflected back into the tissues — acts as if it were a completely new sound pulse generated by the transducer and produces a further echo train replicating the original echo pattern. Every structure in the scan will be repeated throughout the scan at intervals which are multiples of the

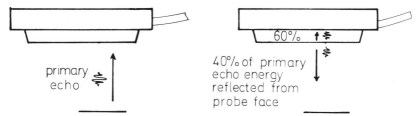

Fig. 1.19 The probe has a different acoustic impedance to tissue. This causes a large proportion of the energy in an echo to be returned to the tissues as a secondary pulse.

distance between the probe and the structure producing the primary echo (Fig. 1.20). Fortunately, in practice, the majority of reverberant echoes are too weak to be registered by the equipment, but become troublesome if the primary echo is very strong, or if the sensitivity of the equipment is increased, and the reverberation thereby displayed.

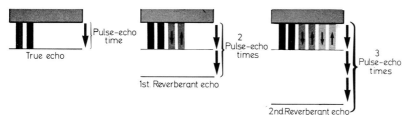

Fig. 1.20 A secondary pulse travelling over the same path as the primary pulse gives rise to a reverberant echo at twice the depth of the primary echo. Further reverberations may occur so that equispaced artefactual echoes are registered on the scan.

Reverberation, of the kind we have been discussing, is seen particularly when there is a distinct boundary running parallel to the probe face, such as the anterior wall of the bladder (Fig. 1.21). A reverberant echo can often be distinguished by the simple expedient of slightly pressing the transducer up and down on the patient's skin. A small reduction of the distance between the probe and an echogenic surface causes a reverberant echo to move closer to the primary echo position and all subsequent reverberations to bunch together because of the reduced length of the sound path. Thus, as the probe is pushed up and down, the spacing between reverberant echoes appears to contract and expand quite markedly.

Of course, reverberation may occur within a structure completely independently from the probe. Generally a strong pulse of sound reflected from a very distinct boundary causes multiple echoes to occur between it and small structures just proximal to it (Fig. 1.22). This type of reverberation normally appears as a haze of echoes distal to the strong reflector. It can be particularly troublesome when the reverberation arises from the anterior uterine wall and may, on occasion, give a very strong impression of an anterior placenta. When an anterior placenta is only suggested by the echo pattern, rather than being absolutely obvious, great care must be taken to investigate the entire uterus to ensure that the scan is not being misinterpreted (Fig. 1.23).

OTHER TYPES OF REAL-TIME EQUIPMENT

In order to understand some of the more sophisticated equipment available we must remind ourselves briefly of some elementary physics. Fig. 1.24 depicts two small sources of sound. The high pressure regions around them are indicated as circles, the areas between the circles representing low pressure regions. If both sound sources produce waves of similar frequency and

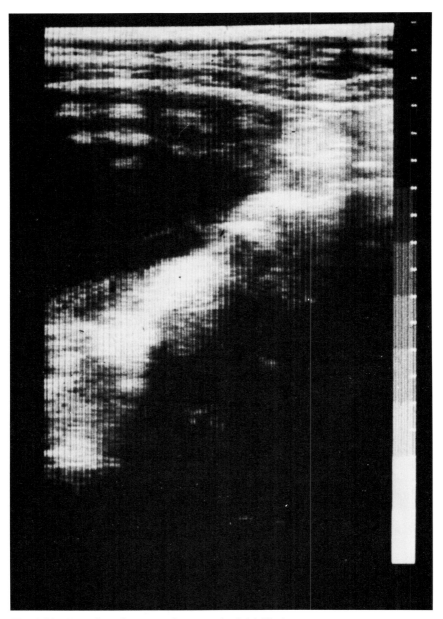

Fig. 1.21 Reverberations are often seen in fluid-filled structures such as the urinary bladder. Care must be taken to avoid misdiagnosis of these areas in the scan. Notice how the reverberation follows the contour of the primary echo.

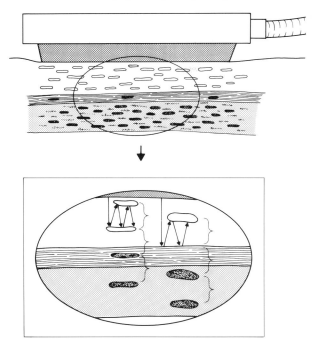

Fig. 1.22   Reverberation is also generated within tissues and is generally seen beyond a strongly reflecting surface such as the anterior uterine wall. Echoes from such a surface are reflected back to it by nearby inhomogeneities. The effect is to form a 'cloud' of echoes similar to those generated by the tissue above the reflector.

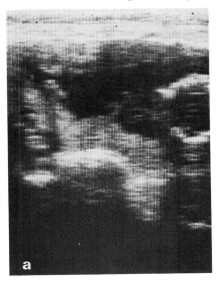
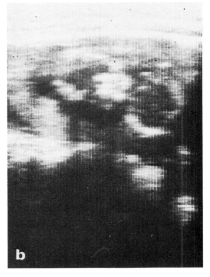

Fig. 1.23a   This longitudinal scan shows a posterior placenta extending into the fundus on the left and apparently having an anterior component. That this component was a tissue reverberation artefact became clear shortly afterwards when **b** the fetus moved and the fetal trunk is seen merging into the 'placental' echoes.

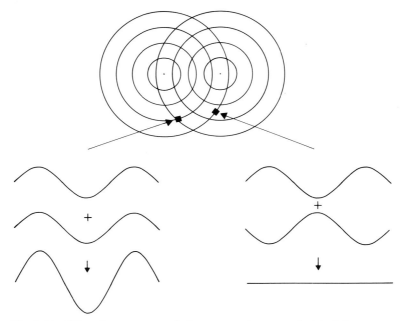

Fig. 1.24   When the pressure peaks in two sound waves coincide (left) then constructive interference occurs. When a peak coincides with a trough then destructive interference occurs.

amplitude then there will be a doubling of pressure at points where the high pressure regions cross. At points where a high pressure region coincides with a low pressure region the pressure waves will cancel out. These phenomena are known as constructive and destructive interference.

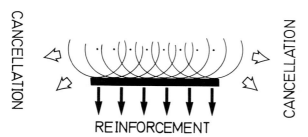

Fig. 1.25   Diagram illustrating the production of a beam.

Fig. 1.25 shows how a number of point sources — all radiating together, in phase and with similar amplitude — produce a region of constructive interference tangental to the wavefronts, whilst in other directions destructive interference occurs. Such interference results in beam formation. A flat-faced transducer may be considered to be made up of a very large number of point sources packed together and radiating in unison. By drawing sufficient wavefronts, the beam patterns in Fig. 1.26 could be predicted. This type of construction, known as Huygens Wave Construction Principle, enables us to derive the beam shape produced by any idealized source radiating continuous-wave ultrasound.

When pulses of sound are produced the situation is much more complex, but the simple model is always helpful. In Fig. 1.26 we see how this principle

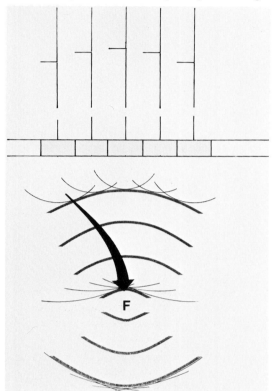

Fig. 1.26 By triggering the outer elements before the inner elements in a transducer group the wavefronts are produced so that the tangental line is curved. This gives rise to a focussing effect and the technique is called dynamic focussing.

of the pulse energy being concentrated along a direction tangential to the wavefronts may be used to our advantage. If, instead of energizing a number of sequential elements simultaneously, we were to trigger the innermost elements fractionally after the outermost elements, then the wavefront is focussed, the depth of the focal region being related to the delay between the trigger pulses. This type of focussing is known as 'dynamic focussing' and is frequently used to improve the beam characteristics. It may not be immediately obvious that the focussing may be performed on the received beam as well as on the pulse which is generated by the transducers. However, the process may be inverted by allowing the echo signal at each transducer element to be delayed by an appropriate amount with respect to the others before the signals are added together for display. In this way, focussing is achieved during reception of echoes. By focussing the beam at one distance when the pulse is generated and at a number of different distances when the echoes are received, an extended focal region may be achieved.

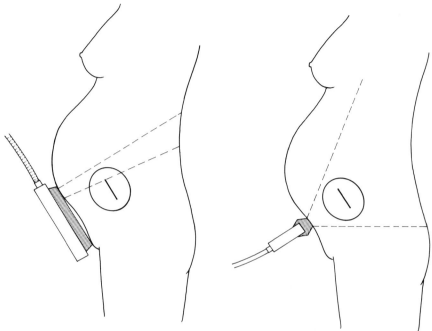

Fig. 1.27   The contours of the patient may make contact between the linear array probe and the skin difficult to achieve. A device producing a fan-shaped scan may be advantageous for reliable access.

One problem with real-time linear arrays is that their long and straight construction does not always allow an easy fit to the contours of the patient and occasionally an air gap appears underneath the probe. The difference in density between air and the patient is large and so virtually all the sound (99.99%) is reflected at an air/patient interface which results in the obliteration of the scan in this region. It is for this reason that a coupling medium such as water-soluble gel is applied to the patient's abdomen. An alternative approach is to use a much smaller transducer which produces a 'fan beam' scan (Fig. 1.27). One method of achieving this result is to use a simple mechanical device in which a number of transducers (normally four or five) are mounted on the edge of a rotating wheel. The wheel is usually covered by a flexible membrane, and the small intervening space is filled with oil. Each time a transducer points down into the tissues it is energized and receives echoes (Fig. 1.28). Fig. 1.29 shows the type of scan produced. Two major

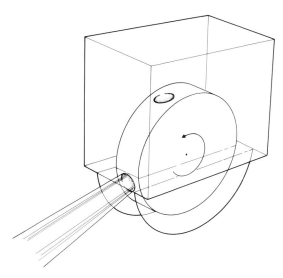

Fig. 1.28 A rotating wheel with transducers mounted on the edge has been successfully produced commercially. The sound beam is produced and echoes received by the transducer adjacent to the acoustic window.

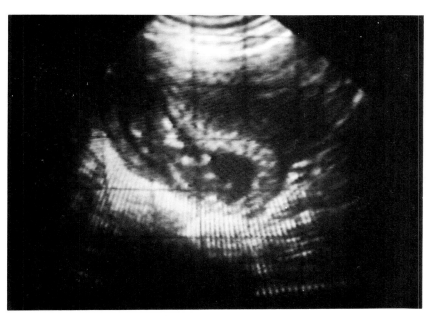

Fig. 1.29 A transverse scan taken with a rotating transducer assembly (spinner). The scan shows an eighteen-week fetus facing the placenta. (By kind permission of Prof. I. Donald and E.M.I. (Medical) Ltd.)

problems are, firstly, that proximal structures not directly in front of the probe are not visualized. Secondly, the extended spacing of the timebase lines in the distal region of the scan causes loss of detail. A significant advantage is that a single, large transducer element can produce a better beam profile than the multiple elements of an array.

All mechanical devices are subject to wear and require regular maintenance. After a time, the coupling which selects the transducer to be triggered is likely to become 'noisy', and problems due to air bubbles in the oil-filled space may also occur. For these reasons, the phased array was produced which performs a similar function to the rotating wheel but uses an electronic technique. Again, the designers have made use of the principle of the pulse energy being concentrated along the line tangental to wavefronts generated by the individual transducer elements. By producing a very short, regular delay between the trigger pulses applied to a group of elements, the beam will not be propagated along the normal beam axis but at an angle to it (Fig. 1.30).

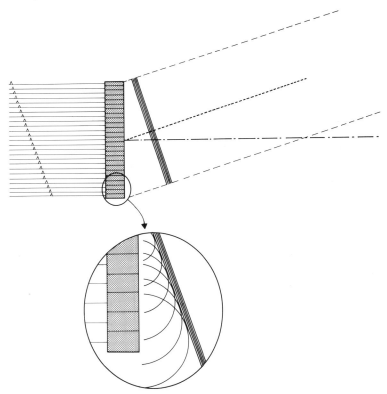

Fig. 1.30   A fan-shaped scan may be produced electronically with a phased array probe. Some 20 thin transducer elements are packed together to form a composite probe about 2 cm across. By triggering the elements in sequence the tangent to the wavefronts makes an angle with the probe face and the beam is directed at an angle to the probe axis.

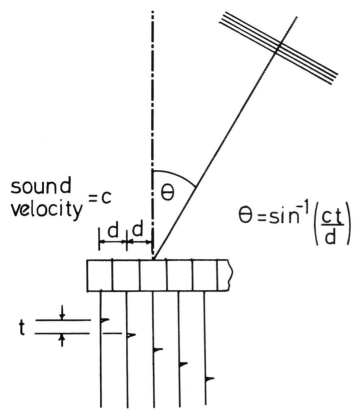

sound
velocity = c

$\theta = \sin^{-1}\left(\dfrac{ct}{d}\right)$

Fig. 1.31 The angle between the beam and the probe axis depends upon the spacing of the elements d, the speed of sound in the body c, and the time delay t, between the triggering of each element. By altering the only variable (t) between each pulse the beam can be swept through a complete range of angles.

Fig. 1.31 shows that the angle which the beam makes with the probe face is related to the speed of sound and the separation of the elements — both of which are constants — and to the time delay between the trigger pulses. Thus, by changing the time delay between successive pulses, the beam can be steered through a series of angles to produce the effect achieved by using the mechanical rotating wheel (popularly referred to as the 'Spinner'). One British version of this equipment is made by EMI. The small size of the probe is obvious (Fig. 1.32).

CONCLUSION

The development of real-time scanners is still in its infancy and we can expect to see improvements in resolution and picture clarity, and a reduction in size

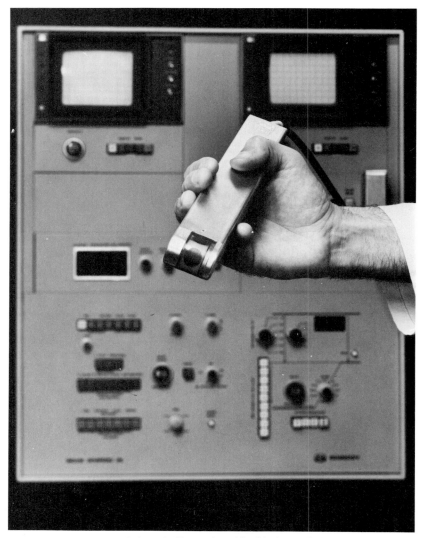

Fig. 1.32   The E.M.I. 'Spinner'. (Reproduced by kind permission of E.M.I. (Medical) Ltd.).

and cost. However, some of the difficulties we have described are inherent in the technique and the user must make the effort to understand possible artefacts which may be caused by these difficulties if he is to avoid the embarrassment, or worse, of making a false diagnosis.

CHAPTER 2

Clinical potential of real-time ultrasound

S. Campbell & D. J. Little

There is no doubt that the development of the real-time scanner has transformed prenatal care. Ultrasound is now no longer a diagnostic test applied to a few pregnancies regarded on clinical grounds as being at risk. It can now be used to screen all pregnancies and should be regarded as an integral part of prenatal care. As a consequence many obstetricians now find themselves in a position of purchasing such equipment, and the twenty or more commercially available real-time scanners (McGraphics 1979) bear testament to the intense commercial interest being taken in these machines for obstetric monitoring. It seems appropriate therefore to begin by discussing the essential features of a real-time scanner. Many machines being produced at the moment lack some of these prerequisites and some manufacturers quote a price with essential features as additional extras, thus misleading the purchaser as to the true financial outlay involved.

CONSIDERATIONS WHEN PURCHASING REAL-TIME EQUIPMENT

1 Linear array or sector scanner.
2 Grey scale and resolution.
3 Freeze-frame.
4 Measuring systems.
5 A-scan and TM facility.
6 Scale expansion and ergonomics.
7 Portability.
8 Video recording and photography.
9 Cost: hardware, maintenance contract, running costs.

1 The first consideration must be to determine which type of real-time system to purchase. Is it wise to play safe with one of the many linear array scanners at present available, or would one of the mechanical or phased array

sector scanners be more suitable for obstetric examination? We will discuss here only the mechanical sector scanner, as the phased array scanner appears to have several disadvantages which make it unsuitable for obstetric scanning. It is much more expensive, bulkier and less portable than the mechanical version. Furthermore the first 3 cm are 'lost' due to blanking out to overcome reverberation problems, and, currently, echo resolution does not seem to be superior to that of the mechanical sector scanners. There is little doubt that the smaller transducer of the mechanical sector machines appears to confer considerable advantages over the larger and more cumbersome linear array transducers. With the latter type it is often impossible to angle the beam across the parietal eminences if the head is in either the direct occipito-anterior or occipito-posterior position, or is deeply engaged. This is less of a problem with a smaller sector scanner transducer, and the 'lining up' of the fetal crown–rump length (CRL) or biparietal diameter (BPD) in early pregnancy is usually a quick and simple exercise with the 'spinner'. Furthermore, if the sector scanner can give 90° or 180° sector images in late pregnancy, this can be useful when circumference measurements of the head and abdomen are desired. With the linear array transducers the application of the complete length of the array to the maternal abdomen in late pregnancy is frequently impossible in the transverse plane due to the convexity of the

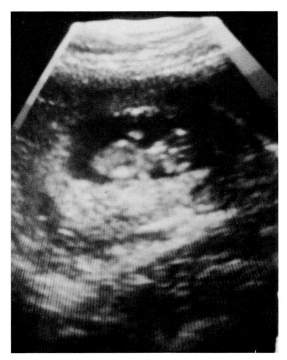

Fig. 2.1   Echogram of fetal crown–rump length taken with a mechanical sector scanner (Combison 100).

maternal abdomen, so that a complete outline of the fetal head or abdomen cannot be obtained. The resolution of the mechanical sector scanners is far better than that of linear arrays in early pregnancy, and is superior even to that of the large static compound scanners as movement artefact is avoided (Fig. 2.1).

The mechanical sector scanners, therefore, are extremely valuable for early CRL measurements and for the early detection of multiple pregnancy. They are extremely good at demonstrating limb length and may have a potential in the future for the early diagnosis of cardiac abnormalities. The 5-transducer systems are flicker-free and can therefore demonstrate fetal heart activity as early as 8 weeks menstrual age. Those with less than 5 transducers have a flicker which makes it difficult to identify fetal heart action during the very early weeks of pregnancy.

The disadvantages of the mechanical sector scanners become more apparent in the third trimester of pregnancy. There are problems with poor lateral resolution in the deeper layers, and acoustic shadowing is often severe when the fetal spine is anterior. A disturbing finding is a consistent curvature of the midline echo of the fetal head in late pregnancy. This is at present inexplicable but may possibly be a feature of beam width. Finally, there is a problem of orientation; a relatively small rotatory, lateral or antero-posterior movement can cause major alterations in the plane of the scan. This can cause difficulties in orientation for even experienced operators.

On balance, therefore, for most obstetric purposes, the linear array scanners would seem to be preferable and further discussion of real-time scanning will relate to the linear array systems.

2   The most important consideration of all when purchasing a machine is the provision of a high resolution picture with good grey scaling. Without good picture quality it does not matter what additional facilities are available — the machine is not worth purchasing. The best resolution is undoubtedly obtained with transducers which have some kind of electronic focussing. Grey scale is less easy to quantify but is readily appreciated subjectively; this is a good reason for insisting on trying out the apparatus on patients before deciding to purchase. A good test of resolution and grey scaling is to perform a fetal CRL measurement between 8 and 12 weeks menstrual age (Fig. 2.2). With the best scanners, CRL measurements are easily obtained and fetal heart movements easily identifiable. Unfortunately some scanners being marketed at the moment give blotchy pictures with poor resolution, so that it is difficult to distinguish the early fetus from other echo-producing structures. Other tests of picture quality are to identify the fetal cerebral ventricular system between 16 and 20 weeks, to obtain clear outlines of the fetal abdominal circumference between 14 and 20 weeks and of fetal renal outlines between 18 and 22 weeks.

3   An important feature which has not yet been incorporated into all real-time scanners is a freeze-frame. The advantages of this facility are obvious; with a rapidly moving fetus it is often difficult to view a particular organ

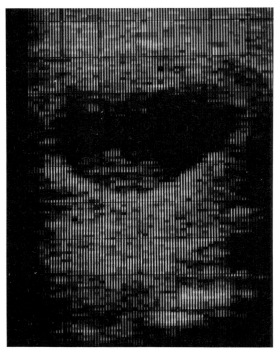

Fig. 2.2 Echogram of fetal crown-rump length taken with linear array real-time scanner (ADR).

or section of the fetus for any length of time, and the ability to freeze the picture when an optimal section has been obtained permits detailed study. It will also allow on-screen measurements of a particular diameter or circumference which would otherwise be time-consuming or inaccurate with a moving picture. For example, a head in the occipito-posterior position will often move into a suitable position for measuring before reverting to the unfavourable one again. The ability to freeze the image in the optimal position will save an enormous amount of time and permit more accurate placement of the caliper spots. One should be able to zoom the image on the freeze-frame without loss of resolution, and it is important that there should be no loss of grey scale on freeze; there is a tendency towards a more bistable image with some freeze-frame systems.

4   Having achieved an optimal frozen image it is important to have an accurate and easily applicable on-screen measuring system. Most real-time scanners provide a facility for measuring the BPD or CRL. The best systems are omnidirectional, which means that the calipers can be moved onto interfaces in any axis from the oblique to the vertical. Ideally, however, on-screen measuring should also include area and circumference (perimeter) measurements of the fetal head and abdomen, for these have been shown to be of great value is assessing fetal weight (Campbell & Wilkin 1975) and growth (Camp-

bell & Thoms 1977). At the present such measurements are usually obtained by applying a planimeter or curvimeter (map measurer) to the images on polaroid photographs, but this technique has inherent inaccuracies and is very expensive. It is now possible to purchase on-screen measuring systems which obviate the difficulties described above and some manufacturers have incorporated these into their real-time systems. This is either done by 'joy sticking' a caliper spot round the outline to be measured, or by tracing the spot round with a light pen. The latter system would seem to be preferable as control of the caliper spot is greater, but both systems are a considerable improvement on measurements made from polaroid photographs. Linear dimensions can also be measured accurately by on-screen systems. Having obtained a digital readout of the appropriate measurement, a microprocessor built into the caliper unit can be used to calculate the gestational age, fetal weight and growth rate by reference to stored normal data. This sort of facility lightens the work of the operator and greatly increases patient throughput. Two manufacturers provide these facilities which make a very attractive package for the purchaser.

5   The most precise method of measuring any linear dimension is by A-scan, and some manufacturers provide an A-scan display either on a separate cathode ray tube or across one margin of the real-time display. While acknowledging the increased precision of the A-scan measurement, it is likely that most operators will find that this leads to delay and thus the main advantage of real-time measurements — which is speed — will be lost. On-screen measurements with the present caliper systems are sufficiently accurate for most clinical situations. Likewise the provision of a TM display has no advantages in the routine clinical situation, although it may be useful in the assessment of fetal cardiac output.

6   The ability to expand the scale of the image without significant loss of definition is important, and it should always be remembered that the larger the image the more accurate will be the measurement of fetal size, especially if the measurements are made on-screen. Zoom on 'write' is the ideal method of enlarging the display, for there will be no loss of inherent resolution. Zoom on 'read' is more common, but detail is not enhanced by making the scan display bigger. Scale expansion frequently means that a region of interest is no longer visible and controls for re-centering such an area should be easily accessible. Many machines make this a difficult manoeuvre and the ergonomics of the control panel should be carefully assessed when buying a machine.

7   Most advertisements for real-time scanners stress that their system is portable, but only a few can be picked up and carried like a suitcase. Most of the others can be pushed around on a trolley, and for most purchasers this will be acceptable. However, for doctors, who wish to move their real-time scanner between hospitals or antenatal clinics, a truly portable machine is essential. The quality of the trolleys that are provided with real-time equipment should be carefully assessed for many are flimsy and are unlikely

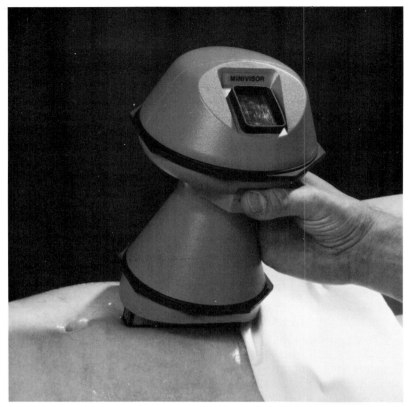

Fig. 2.3   Hand-held, battery-operated linear array real-time scanner.

to withstand the considerable wear that occurs when the apparatus is frequently moved between departments. If the purchaser wishes to make video recordings then the trolley should also be able to contain such equipment.

The ultimate in portability is the new battery-operated, hand-held real-time scanner (Fig. 2.3). Many doctors tend to regard this piece of equipment as a gimmick, and it must be admitted that the resolution and grey scale of the images are, as yet, inferior to that of the best conventional real-time scanners. Furthermore, the small area of the abdomen covered by the transducer and the small screen are difficulties which are initially disconcerting. I believe, however, that this type of machine may have a very useful function. To achieve their full potential these small scanners should probably be used by all trained obstetricians and midwives. Thus, in the antenatal clinic, they can be used to diagnose multiple pregnancy and provide immediate information on the presentation and position of the fetus, the placental site and fetal heart activity. The machine can be taken from patient to patient in the antenatal clinic, thus increasing the likelihood of picking up problems that may not find their way to a more formal ultrasound examination. In the labour ward it will allow the on-duty registrar to elucidate emergency problems occurring in labour. Finally, I believe it will make the use of real-time scanning and the interpretation of ultrasound images part of a specialist's training which must provide benefits in a more widespread and intelligent use of ultrasound in the future.

8   If measurements are to be made from polaroid photographs the primary screen must be used. This can lead to difficulties if a TV camera is used simultaneously to provide a video recording. Polaroid photographs have the advantage of being immediately available for measuring but are expensive (30 pence per exposure), show inferior grey scaling and are less tolerant of alterations in image brightness than 70 mm or 35 mm film. A slave monitor can be used for 35 mm and 70 mm photography, and this provides high quality images at low cost — i.e. between 2 and 4 pence per exposure. Non-portable systems such as multiformat imagers are not relevant to real-time ultrasound. With non-instant photography, image identification requires some method of recording patient data on the film. Some real-time scanners have the facility to display the patient's record number via the video system. If this is not possible an add-on electronic character generator will be required.

Video recording is most useful, particularly in abnormal cases and for teaching purposes. It is also essential if studies of fetal respiratory movement, cardiac activity and motor activity are being made. A TV camera is widely used to provide the video signal but the best recordings are obtained by direct video. This is a digital electronic process which provides a TV picture directly from the electronic information generated by the real-time machine. Video recorders can be used to record still images in the single frame mode. It is possible to provide several thousand images per tape but recalling individual frames at a later date is cumbersome.

9   Due to intense competition the price of real-time scanners has remained remarkably stable despite inflation and despite the increasing number of extras that are now available. Potential purchasers should determine whether items such as extra TV monitors, freeze-frame, electronic calipers and character generators are included in the basic price. A maintenance contract should also be negotiated at the time of purchase. Some manufacturers are much more reasonable in this regard than others, though at the same time the purchaser should enquire as to the quality of service provided by the manufacturer's local agent and the reliability of the equipment. Running costs are of great importance. A system which requires the taking of polaroid photographs for area and circumference measurements will be expensive. For example, in 1978, the bill for polaroid photographs in the Obstetric Ultrasound Department at King's College Hospital was in the region of £8000. In general the price of real-time scanners varies from £9000 to £18 000, but as the more expensive machines may provide better facilities for taking measurements and superior image quality, cost alone should not dominate the decision as to which is the best buy. In the UK economic considerations have too often determined which static B-scanner will be purchased. Unfortunately, in the past, the gantry which held the transducer often was unsuitable for obstetric measurements, and as a consequence the machine was confined to some far corner of the hospital, unused and gathering dust. These false economies should be resisted; ultrasound, when used properly, will not only help to reduce perinatal mortality and morbidity, but will also save money by reducing the number of unnecessary admissions and inductions of labour. An initial outlay of an extra few thousand pounds can make sense in economic terms if the clinical results are significantly improved.

CLINICAL ROLE FOR REAL-TIME SCANNING

Real-time scanning has 'burst' on the clinical scene within a short space of time and it will be several years before the true place of this new development is known. Despite the fact that our opinions will certainly alter over the next few years, we will nevertheless try to chart the future role for real-time scanning. Real-time scanners are small, cheap, mobile and easy to apply; they provide rapid ultrasound assessment and measurement and we believe can be used efficiently by a range of reasonably intelligent personnel (doctors, nurses, technicians) after a short period of training. For these reasons we believe that in future they will be placed in the antenatal clinic which will make the routine screening of obstetric patients easier and will obviate the need for the usual facilities that are required by ultrasound departments such as waiting and changing rooms, receptionists and extra nurses. Real-time scanning will have a major role to play in the examination of the pregnant uterus before 12 weeks gestation. CRL measurements for dating can be performed from 7 weeks with good accuracy and this is especially true of the mechanical sector scanner (see Fig. 2.1).

Fetal movement and heart activity can also be recognized from 9 weeks onwards (and occasionally as early as 7 weeks) so that the initial assessment of patients with threatened abortion will usually be undertaken with real-time machines. However, the definitive diagnosis of embryonic death should still be made with the static B-scanner, certainly until the reliability of the real-time machines has been more clearly established. The early diagnosis of multiple pregnancy before 12 weeks by the process of 'counting the sacs' should also be reliably made by real-time scanning (it should be remembered, however, that after 10 weeks the ability to determine the correct number of sacs is frequently undermined by an overlapping of the sacs in a single plane).

Routine scanning of every pregnant patient before 12 weeks may soon become part of our antenatal programme and certainly it will provide early and accurate dating of the fetus. However, we believe that routine screening between 16 and 18 weeks (our present scheme) is more useful for the following reasons:

1   BPD measurements are easily obtained for dating the pregnancy.

Although the prediction of fetal age may be marginally less precise when compared with early CRL measurements (by ± 4 days) this is insignificant in clinical terms.

2   Dating measurements can also be performed from a measurement of abdominal circumference; this is a useful check on the BPD prediction and adds confidence to the assessment.

3   Fetal measurements can be obtained without the need for a full maternal bladder which is necessary in pre-12 week measurements; filling the bladder of each new booking patient at the antenatal clinic can be time consuming and disruptive to clinic routine.

4   Early diagnosis of multiple pregnancy is more easily made by counting the fetal heads and bodies.

5   The placenta can be localized and a group of patients with 'low lying' placentae recognized. This group of patients will be at high risk of having a placenta praevia (Campbell & Little 1977), but it should be stressed that it is impossible definitely to recognize placenta praevia at this stage. However, it is reassuring to visualize the placenta in the fundus of the uterus and, when this has been identified, a placenta praevia is excluded.

6   Gross fetal abnormalities such as anencephaly can be reliably diagnosed. Although we have recognized spina bifida at 17 weeks by real-time scanning it is unlikely that this technique will be used routinely to screen out spina bifida at the present. With the improvements in ultrasound equipment that are anticipated, a comparative study of routine real-time scanning and maternal serum alphafetoprotein will be interesting. Hydrocephalus is manifested at 16–18 weeks by enlargement of the ventricles and not of the cranium (Campbell 1978), and we have recognized both this condition and exomphalos on the real-time display. Although such abnormalities are rare, the occasional recognition of such defects is further justification for using 16–18 weeks as the time for routine screening. As maternal serum alphafetoprotein is also performed at this time, the examinations can conveniently be combined.

A second routine screening examination at 32 weeks to obtain a fetal abdomen circumference measurement would also be of value in identifying the small-for-dates fetus. We have previously predicted (Campbell & Wilkin 1975) that abdominal circumference measurements taken at 32 weeks with a static B-scanner will detect 87% of small-for-dates fetuses with only a 1% incidence of false-positive diagnosis. The accuracy of real-time measurements for this purpose has yet to be determined, but our initial experience suggests that routine screening by this method would be a significant advance in the detection of the small-for-dates fetus.

Amniocentesis is most safely performed under the guidance of ultrasound and real-time scanners are ideal for this purpose, for the placental margin can usually be clearly identified. Most doctors now believe that amniocentesis should be performed after ultrasound placental localization, but few actually perform the procedure coincidentally with the ultrasound examination. This we believe is a mistake because it is possible to identify an accessible pool of liquor which may not be present if amniocentesis is performed some hours later. Indeed, we frequently find that, because of rotation of the uterus with fetal movement or maternal bladder filling, a 'safe' site marked on the maternal abdomen may be situated over the placenta or fetus some hours later. In future, amniocentesis is likely to be performed in the antenatal clinic under the guidance of real-time scanning. Similarly real-time scanning will also have an important part to play in making fetoscopy a safer and more reliable procedure, and in our department, ultrasound-guided fetoscopy is used to obtain pure samples of fetal blood from the insertion of the umbilical cord (Mibashan *et al* 1979). This is already enlarging the scope of prenatal diagnosis and is further discussed in Chapter 5. Ultrasound-guided fetoscopy can be used to diagnose fetal defects which are beyond the resolving power of ultrasound, but it is likely that some fetal abnormalities will only be recognized with the help of real-time scanning. For instance, limb reduction deformities are extremely difficult to recognize with static B-scanners because of the constraints imposed by the gantry, but, with practice, a full limb length can usually be obtained with the real-time apparatus. The chambers of the heart and valves can clearly be seen from 18 weeks onwards especially with mechanical sector scanners, and with intensive study it may be possible to diagnose certain congenital abnormalities prenatally.

Real-time scanning has opened up a completely new dimension for fetal study — i.e. monitoring of fetal activity and behaviour. The two parameters which are under close study are fetal respiratory movements and fetal motor activity during the third trimester, and these are being used as an index of fetal well-being. In our own laboratory we have been measuring the percentage incidence of fetal respiratory movements and fetal trunk movements as these can both be assessed on a single transverse section of the upper fetal abdomen. Preliminary results are presented in Chapter 10. It is important to realize that, in the normal fetus, there is a wide variation in the incidence of both these parameters in any 30-minute study period, and it is unlikely that fetal breathing or even fetal motor activity will be the definitive test if such an entity exists. It is likely, however, that a physical profile of fetal dynamics will be produced which will assist in determining the optimal time for delivery or the need for antenatal therapy. The reaction of the fetus to various stimuli such as maternal CO_2 inhalation, glucose loading or even audible sound may also help to identify an at-risk group. For such studies to become popular, however, fetal activity will need to be automatically recorded by the machine as occurs with antenatal and intrapartum cardiotocography. This will be difficult with fetal respiratory movement for, even when generalized motor activity is not occurring, the upper fetal abdomen can move rhythmically in response to the maternal diaphragm, maternal aorta and fetal heart. At the present, only the human brain can distinguish between these various components of fetal movement. Probably the best approach to this problem would be automated perimeter tracking; the image of the fetal chest or abdomen is registered in digital format and any alterations can be continuously monitored.

New developments in understanding fetal physiology are also opening up as a result of real-time studies of the fetal heart and blood vessel movement. The Dublin group (Fitzgerald & Drumm 1977) have produced peak velocity profiles from the umbilical vessels, while others (Winsberg 1972, Wladimiroff *et al* 1979) are attempting to estimate fetal cardiac output from volume changes in the chambers of the heart, combining real-time and TM information for this purpose. In the future fetal circulatory changes resulting from pre-eclampsia, diabetes, ante-partum haemorrhage and other complications of pregnancy should almost certainly be measurable. When taken with fetal activity, antenatal heart monitoring and serial measurement of fetal size, this will give a detailed physical profile of the fetus which should supplant biochemical studies as a means of assessing fetal well-being.

CLINICAL ROLE FOR STATIC B-SCANNING

It is unlikely that static B-scanning will be superseded completely by real-time scanning in at least the foreseeable future. Although a longitudinal section of the fetal spine can be easily obtained with the real-time scanner it should be remembered that the diagnosis of spina bifida can only be made with certainty on a transverse section of the fetal spine (Campbell *et al* 1975), and a static B-scan machine gives superior cross-sectional images of the spine. This advantage lies in the ability to compound the scan with a static system (thus enabling axial resolution to be utilized on interfaces in the vertical axis) and this superiority is also evident when outlining fetal cerebral ventricles or fetal kidneys between 16 and 22 weeks' gestation. The early detection of fetal ascites is also best done with the static scanners.

Measurement of the biparietal diameter, head circumference and abdomen circumference is, in experienced hands, more accurate by static B-scan measurement, and serial weekly or bi-weekly measurements to assess fetal growth are ideally made by this method in late pregnancy. Under normal circumstances fetal growth is slow at this time, and its measurement must be performed by the most precise method available. Finally, accurate identification of the lower extremity of the placenta can occasionally be difficult with real-time scanners, as the margin frequently runs in the vertical axis, and the ability to compound the scan is essential when this problem obtains.

REFERENCES

CAMPBELL S. (1968) An improved method of fetal cephalometry by ultrasound. *J. Obstet. Gynaecol. Br. Commonw.* **75,** 568.

CAMPBELL S. (1976) Fetal growth. In *Fetal Physiology and Medicine*, eds. R. W. Beard and P. Nathanleiz. W. B. Saunders, Philadelphia.

CAMPBELL S. (1978) Early prenatal diagnosis of fetal abnormality by ultrasound B-scanning. *Proceedings of the 3rd European Conference on Prenatal Diagnosis of Genetic Disorders*, eds. J.-D. Murken, S. Stengel-Rutkowski and E. Schwinger, p. 183. Ferdinand Enke, Stuttgart.

CAMPBELL S. & KURJAK A. (1972) Comparison between urinary oestrogen assay and serial ultrasonic cephalometry in assessment of fetal weight. *Br. J. Obstet. Gynaecol.* **82,** 689.

CAMPBELL S. & LITTLE D. J. (1977) Clinical potential of latest equipment. Symposium on the Current Status of Fetal Heart Fate Monitoring in Ultrasound in Obstetrics. *Proceedings of Scientific Meeting of the Royal College of Obstetricians and Gynaecologists*, eds. S. Campbell and R. W. Beard, p. 183.

CAMPBELL S. & NEWMAN G. B. (1971) Growth of the Fetal Biparietal Diameter during Pregnancy. *J. Obstet. Gynaecol. Br. Commonw.* **78,** 513.

CAMPBELL S., PRYSE-DAVIES J., COLTART T. M., SELLER M. J. & SINGER J. D. (1975) Ultrasound in the diagnosis of spina bifida. *Lancet* i, 1065.

CAMPBELL S. & THOMS A. (1977) Ultrasound measurement of the fetal head to abdomen circumference ratio in the assessment of growth retardation. *Br. J. Obstet. Gynaecol.* **84,** 165.

CAMPBELL S. & WILKIN D. (1975) Ultrasonic measurement of the fetal abdominal circumference in the estimation of fetal weight. *Br. J. Obstet. Gynaecol.* **82,** 689.

COOPERBERG P. L., GHOW T., KITE V. & AUSTIN S. (1976) *J. Clin. Ultrasound.* **4,** 421.

DAVISON J. M., LIND T., FARR V. & WHITTINGHAM T. A. (1973) The limitations of ultrasonic fetal cephalometry. *J. Obstet. Gynaecol. Br. Commonw.* **80,** 924.

DOCKER M. F. & SETTATREE R. S. (1977) Comparison between linear array real-time ultrasonic scanning and conventional compound scanning in the measurement of the fetal biparietal diameter. *Br. J. Obstet. Gynaecol.* **84,** 924.

FITZGERALD D. E. & DRUMM J. E. (1977) Non-invasive measurement of the human fetal circulation — a new method. *Br. med. J.* ii, 1450.

LUNT R. M. & CHARD T. (1974) Reproducibility of measurement of fetal biparietal diameter by ultrasound cephalometry. *Br. J. Obstet. Gynaecol.* **81,** 682.

McGRAPHICS (1979) *Clinical ultrasound purchasers' catalogue.* 409 So. Sherman, Denver, Colorado, USA.

MIBASHAN R. S., RODECK C. H., THUMPSTON J. K., EDWARDS R. J., SINGER J. D., WHITE J. M. & CAMPBELL S. (1979) Prenatal diagnosis of haemophilia by plasma assay of fetal factors VII and IX. *Lancet*, in Press.

ROBINSON H. P. (1973) Sonar measurement of fetal crown–rump length as a means of assessing maturity in the first trimester. *Br. J. Med.* **4,** 28.

VARMA Y. R. (1973) Prediction of delivery date by ultrasound cephalometry. *J. Obstet. Gynaecol. Br. Commonw.* **80,** 376.

WILLOCKS J., DONALD I., DUGGAN T. C. & DAY N. (1964) Fetal cephalometry by ultrasound. *J. Obstet. Gynaecol. Br. Commonw.* **71,** 11.

WINSBERG F. (1972) Echocardiography of the fetal and newborn heart. *Inv. Radiol.* **7,** 152.

WLADIMIROFF J. W., VOSTERS W. & VLETTER W. (1979) Ultrasonic measurement of fetal cardiac ventricular dimensions. In *Contributions in Gynaecology and Obstetrics*, ed. R. Chef. S. Karger, Basel.

CHAPTER 3

An evaluation of real-time scanning in the first trimester of pregnancy

A. H. Adam & H. P. Robinson

The principal applications of diagnostic ultrasound in early pregnancy are in confirming the presence of a pregnancy within the uterus, in establishing the presence or absence of fetal life, and in the estimation of gestational age. In assessing the place of real-time scanning equipment in early pregnancy, a comparison has inevitably to be made with what is possible using a conventional scanner. However, an evaluation should also be made of any additional information which devolves from its 'real-time' capability.

DETECTION OF INTRA-UTERINE PREGNANCY

Gestation sac

While clinical signs and hormonal assays only infer the presence of a pregnancy in the first trimester, the demonstration of a gestation sac by ultrasound within the uterus from 5 weeks (menstrual age) is definite proof.

In general, lateral resolution using the linear array type of real-time scanner is not as good as that achieved with a conventional scanner. As a result, and in the authors' experience using linear array equipment, it has not been possible to distinguish the fetus with certainty from much before 9 weeks gestational age (Fig. 3.1), although the gestation sac may itself be visualized from 7 weeks. With future developments such as dynamic focussing, lateral resolution should be improved thereby allowing the delineation of smaller structures. Thus the detection of fetal echoes should be possible from an earlier stage.

This limitation does not apply to the mechanical or rotating transducer such as the 'spinner', where the gestation sac can be visualized from 5 weeks and the presence of the fetal pole can be detected from 6 to 7 weeks (Fig. 3.2). This compares favourably with the capabilities of good conventional equipment.

In the context of this section, a twin pregnancy may be diagnosed with either the linear array or the 'spinner' types of real-time equipment from early

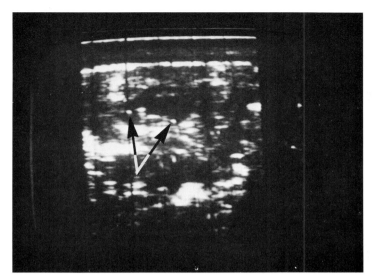

Fig. 3.1   Pregnancy at $8\frac{1}{2}$ weeks scanned using a linear array real-time equipment (Diagnostic Sonar, System 85). Scale = 1:2.
The arrows show the position of the electronic calipers at either end of the fetus, allowing measurement of its crown–rump length (CRL = 22 mm).

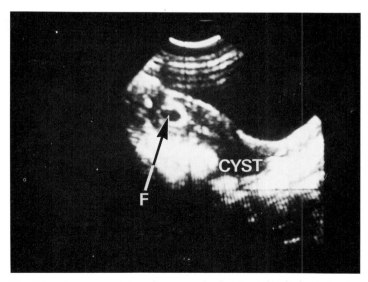

Fig. 3.2   Pregnancy at 6 weeks scanned using a mechanical rotating transducer (E.M.I. Nuclear Enterprises Ltd.).
The fetal pole is just visible (indicated by arrow). There is an associated cyst in the Pouch of Douglas.

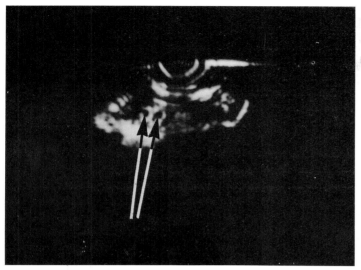

Fig. 3.3 Twin gestation sacs at 6 weeks (mechanical rotating transducer) Scale = 2:5.

in the first trimester, and indeed their capability of allowing a rapid examination of the whole volume of the uterus makes such a diagnosis simpler (Fig. 3.3).

DETECTION AND CONFIRMATION OF FETAL LIFE

In a patient with slight vaginal bleeding or a past history of recurrent abortion, the certain knowledge that the fetus is alive is a prerequisite for the pregnancy to be considered as a continuing one, and, conversely, the certain knowledge that the fetus is dead is the most positive way in which a pregnancy can be classified as a missed abortion. Using ultrasound it has become possible to confirm the presence of fetal life by visualizing the pulsation of the fetal heart from $6\frac{1}{2}$ to 7 weeks (Robinson 1972), by demonstrating movements of the fetus itself from 8 to 9 weeks (Hinselmann 1969), or by recognizing the typical fetal heart 'tones' using an abdominal ultrasound Doppler apparatus from 12 weeks (Callagan *et al* 1964, Johnson *et al* 1965, Jouppila 1971).

Methods of detecting fetal life

The introduction of ultrasonic instruments employing the Doppler principle was the first major step in the detection of fetal life in the first half of pregnancy. The principal limitation to the earlier detection of fetal life (before 12 weeks) using such instruments is the problem of having to search blindly over the whole volume of the pelvis for the fetal heart, an organ which at this stage is a very small structure. This problem was resolved, using conventional B-scan equipment, by a technique where the fetal echo complex is accurately identified on a two-dimensional B or section scan and the fetal echoes closely examined on an expanded unidimensional A-scan (Robinson 1972). Using this technique fetal heart movements can be detected unequivocably at 7 weeks of menstrual age or over.

Using the real-time scanner, a similar two-dimensional B-scan image of the fetus can be obtained. However, since many of the real-time systems do not have A-scan facilities, the method described by Robinson (1972) for conventional equipment is not applicable. Confirmation that the heart is pulsating has then to be made by directly visualizing the moving cardiac structures on the real-time image. The accuracy of detection of these movements is then dependent on the resolution capabilities of the equipment, and on the amplitude of the movements themselves. In practice, a confident diagnosis of fetal life cannot be made from much before 9 to 10 weeks by this method. On the other hand gross fetal body movements are more readily identified, and from 9 weeks onwards such observations are a very useful way of confirming that the fetus is alive. These movements are variable in pattern, ranging from a sudden flick which results in the fetus floating upwards from the bottom of the sac, to wild gyrations which may continue for many seconds.

DIAGNOSIS OF EARLY PREGNANCY FAILURE

Using ultrasound, four distinct groups of early pregnancy failure were described by Robinson (1975a): missed abortions, blighted ova, live abortions, and hydatidiform moles. Two of these, the missed abortions and the blighted ova, rely for their diagnoses on a good resolving power of the ultrasonic equipment and on the experience of the observer.

This statement implies that it is necessary for the clinician to be able to detect a small fetus, should one be present, and to be able to say with complete confidence that fetal heart movements are either present or absent. Since many real-time scanners do not allow the positive recognition of the fetus until 8 weeks or over, and since fetal heart movements cannot be reliably detected until 10 weeks, definite diagnoses of missed abortions and blighted ova should not be made using such equipment until the patient has been pregnant for at least 10 weeks and until several confirmatory examinations have been made. However, as the majority of fetuses in cases of missed abortion die before they reach 10 to 11 weeks size (Robinson 1975a), the use of real-time equipment in this context is limited, at least for the present.

Measurement of the gestation sac diameter may, on the other hand, also be useful, but here serial examinations are even more important.

The remaining two groups, live abortions and hydatidiform moles together constitute only a small proportion of early pregnancy failures. In general, the recognition of a mole should pose no particular problem using a real-time scanner since the volume of the uterus may be rapidly scanned, and since the diagnosis is based on the simple pictorial appearance of the intra-uterine contents rather than on their measurements. The important criteria, as with conventional equipment, are the 'snowstorm' appearance of the intra-uterine echoes and the lack of any recognizable structures.

Live abortions, that is those pregnancies in which the fetus is alive until shortly before spontaneous abortion, cannot be predicted with confidence using either conventional or real-time equipment. However, Reinold has suggested that the study of fetal trunk movements in these cases may prove to be useful. Should this be the case, then real-time equipment would be the apparatus of choice for use in such studies.

FETAL MOVEMENTS

It has long been recognized (Preyer 1885) that fetal movements are present prior to the 17th or 18th week of gestation when they are first discernible by the mother; several authors have reported on the systematic observation of fetal movements *in vitro*, and the characteristics of these movements have been described and related to gestational age and thus to the stage of neurological development (Minkowski 1938, Fitzgerald & Windle 1942). With the introduction of real-time scanning equipment it has become possible to observe early *in vivo* fetal movements (Hofmann *et al* 1961, Hinselmann 1969) thereby enabling more direct information to be obtained about the development of the fetal neuro-muscular system. Similarly it has become possible to study the effect of possible adverse influences on the fetus such as threatened abortion.

Reinold in his extensive studies of this aspect of early pregnancy development, compared the different fetal motor activities observed with the clinical findings and the outcome of pregnancy. He classified fetal movements into a number of well-defined and characteristic patterns: strong and brisk spontaneous movements; slow and sluggish movements; and no movements either spontaneous or induced. In his material, the finding of sluggish fetal movements or absence of spontaneous fetal movements was found to correlate well with later intra-uterine fetal death and abortion.

In a study of normal patients he found that the number of fetal movements during a 5-minute observation period increased with advancing gestational age. He then analysed the results obtained from serial measurements of fetal movements in a group of 14 patients in whom spontaneous abortion occurred. In the majority he found that the number of movements decreased over a period of weeks with their eventual cessation prior to spontaneous abortion (Fig. 3.4). At each examination the viability of the fetus was confirmed by the demonstration of fetal heart activity. Since all 14 pregnancies aborted at 12 weeks of gestational age or later, it seems likely that this technique will be most applicable to 'late live abortions'. However, these observations are less likely to be of value in the much more common problems

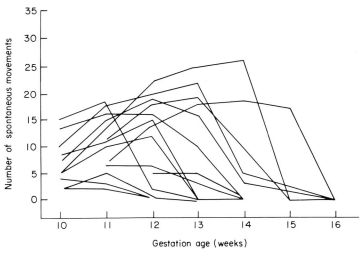

Fig. 3.4 Number of spontaneous fetal movements in 14 pregnancies which aborted spontaneously within a few days of the last examination. At all examinations fetal heart movements had been confirmed. (Reproduced by kind permission from E. Reinold, *Ultrasonics in Early Pregnancy*. S. Karger A.G., Basel.

of early pregnancy, that is the missed abortions and blighted ova which together form the bulk of early pregnancy wastage. In these pregnancies the fetus can almost always be seen to be dead, or the gestation sac seen to be empty or abnormal before 12 weeks using conventional ultrasound techniques (Robinson 1975b).

ESTIMATION OF GESTATIONAL AGE

In view of the importance of an accurate knowledge of gestational age in the management of pregnant patients it has been advocated that all patients should have an ultrasonic scan as early as possible in pregnancy. An early examination is stressed since the predictive value of clinical and ancillary methods of assessing gestational age becomes progressively less reliable.

Gestation sac

In the early weeks of the first trimester the gestation sac is generally spherical but thereafter its shape becomes more variable. Despite these variations, useful clinical information on gestational age may be obtained by measurements of sac diameters (Hellman *et al* 1969, Hoffbauer 1970). In this context, Hoffbauer proposed a simple 'rule of thumb' for clinical purposes: a gestational sac diameter of 2.5 cm is equivalent to 6 weeks; 4 cm equivalent to 8 weeks; and 5 cm equivalent to 10 weeks. Irrespective of which sac measurements are taken — be they diameters, areas or volumes — an estimate of age cannot be given to within any better than ±10 days (Robinson 1975b). This range of potential error is considerably greater than the ±5 days which may be achieved using fetal crown–rump length measurements (Robinson & Fleming 1975). However, since many real-time scanners cannot adequately delineate the fetus before 9 weeks, and since sac measurements can be more easily obtained, this approach to the estimation of gestational age is likely to be the preferred method in at least the earlier part of the first trimester.

Fetal crown–rump length (CRL)

Measurement of the fetal CRL in the first trimester using conventional equipment has been shown to be the most accurate available ancillary method of assessing the age of a pregnancy (Robinson & Fleming 1975).

The practical steps involved in making such measurements with the real-time scanner may be readily adapted from those described for conventional equipment. By moving the hand-held transducer over the abdominal wall, serial longitudinal section scans of the underlying uterus and its contents can be obtained. During this procedure the operator should be able to build up a mental three-dimensional picture of the approximate orientation of the fetus within the gestation sac. A scan along the longitudinal axis of the fetus can then be made and measurements made using the electronic calipers which can be manipulated to any position on the B-scan image. In the absence of such calipers a photograph must be taken and the fetal length measured 'off-line' (Figs. 3.5 & 3.6).

As has been stated by Robinson and Fleming (1975) the reproducibility of the technique is related to a number of potential random errors. These include: operator judgement of the correct axis and the longest length of the fetus; small movements of the fetus and/or mother; and, where relevant, measurement from the photograph. Using real-time equipment fetal movements are readily appreciated and appropriate correction to the plane of scan

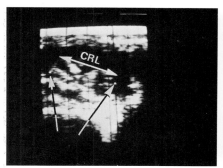 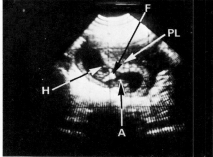

Fig. 3.5 Thirteen-week pregnancy (linear array real-time scanner). Scale = 1:3. The arrows indicate the mechanical calipers at either end of the fetus (CRL = 58 mm).

Fig. 3.6 Twelve-week pregnancy (electronic rotating transducer). Scale = 1:4. F facial area, H Head, A Abdomen, Pl Placenta.

can be made before any measurements are made. The other random errors do not constitute significant practical problems.

In order to assess the difficulties encountered in CRL measurements using a real-time scanner, and the accuracy of the results obtained, 140 patients were examined at a routine antenatal clinic. In scanning an early pregnancy it is usual to examine the patient with a full bladder as this ensures that the uterus is lifted up out of the pelvis and that gas-filled intestines are pushed away. However this is not usually possible in the antenatal clinic since an empty bladder is essential for satisfactory clinical pelvic examinations. Despite this limitation CRL values were obtained from 120 patients. The range of gestation ages of these pregnancies is shown in Table 3.1. For comparative

Table 3.1   Range of gestational age in the 120 patients in whom comparative crown–rump measurements were performed

Gestational age (weeks)	No. patients
8–9	14
10–11	36
12	33
13	27
14	10

purposes measurements were also performed using a conventional B-scanner. A statistical analysis showed that the two sets of measurements were highly correlated ($r = 0.977$).

In 80% of cases, the CRL values using the real-time scanner lay within 5 mm of the value obtained using the conventional scanner (Fig. 3.7). Due to the rapid growth of the fetus in the first trimester, the observed differences in CRL did not result in a discrepancy of more than one week in any patient, when the predicted estimates of gestational age were compared. This applied even in those cases where the observed difference was greater than 5 mm.

CONCLUSION

Real-time scanners perform the majority of tasks demanded of conventional equipment in early pregnancy, albeit that the desired information is often not obtained as early, or with an equal degree of accuracy and reliability. The major limitation of this type of equipment is the inability to make a confident diagnosis of a missed abortion or blighted ovum prior to 10 weeks' gestation. However, with new technical innovations, improving resolution, and increasing experience in using these scanners, this limitation should largely be resolved.

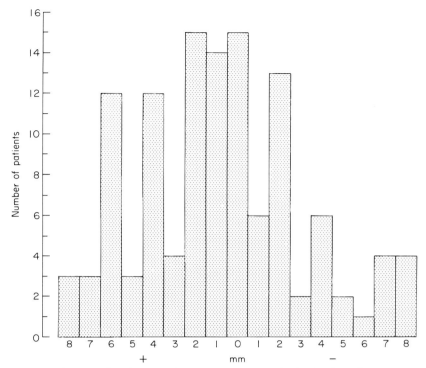

Fig. 3.7 A comparison between CRL measurements obtained using a linear array real-time scanner and those obtained with conventional equipment in a series of 120 patients.

Certain positive advantages are offered by the real-time scanner. Firstly its portability allows the equipment to be used at the antenatal clinic thereby making the logistics of routine early screening for gestational age estimation more feasible; and secondly its real-time function has allowed early fetal movements to be studied, a technique which may well prove to be of prognostic value in patients with late first and early second trimester problems.

REFERENCES

CALLAGAN D. A., ROWLAND T. C. JNR. & GOLDMAN D. E. (1964) Ultrasonic Doppler inspection of the fetal heart. *Obstet. Gynecol.* **23,** 637.

FITZGERALD J. E. & WINDLE W. F. (1942) Some observations on early human fetal movements. *Comp. Neurol.* **76,** 159.

HELLMAN L. M., KOBAYASHI M., FILLISTI L., LAVENHAR M. & CROMB E. (1969) Growth and development of the human fetus prior to the twentieth week of gestation. *Am. J. Obstet. Gynaecol.* **103,** 789.

HINSELMANN M. (1969) Ultraschalldiagnostik in der Geburtshilfe. *Dtsch. Med. Wochenschr.* **94,** 955.

HINSELMANN M. (1969) Ultraschalldiagnostik in der Geburtshilfe. *Gynakologe* **2,** 45.

HOFFBAUER H. (1970) Die Bedeutung der Ultraschalldiagnostik in der Fruhschwanger-schaft. *Electromedica* **3**, 227.

HOFMANN D., HOLLANDER H. J. & WEISER P. (1961) Uber die geburtshilfliche Bedeu-tung der Ultraschalldiagnostik. *Gynaecologia* **164**, 24.

JOHNSON W. L., STEGALL H. F., LEIN J. N. & RUSHMER R. F. (1965) Detection of fetal life in early pregnancy with an ultrasonic Doppler flowmeter. *J. Obstet. Gynecol.* **26**, 305.

JOUPPILA P. (1971) Ultrasound in the diagnosis of early pregnancy and its complications, a comparative study of A, B and Doppler methods. *Acta Obstet. Gynecol. Scand.* **50** (Supplement 15).

MINKOWSKI M. (1938) Neurobiologische Studien am menschlichen Fotus. In *Abder-halden Handbuch der biologischen Arbeitsmethoden*, Abl 5, Teil 5B (Urban and Schwarzenberg) Berlin.

PREYER W. (1885) *Specielle Physiologie des Embryo*. Grieben, Leipzig.

REINOLD E. Ultrasonics in early pregnancy. In *Gynaecology and Obstetrics*, Vol. 1. S. Karger A.G., Basel.

ROBINSON H. P. (1972) Detection of fetal heart movement in the first trimester of preg-nancy using pulsed ultrasound. *Br. med. J.* iv, 466.

ROBINSON H. P. (1975a) The diagnosis of early pregnancy failure by sonar. *Br. J. Obstet. Gynaecol.* **82**, 849.

ROBINSON H. P. (1975b) Gestation sac volumes as determined by sonar in the first tri-mester of pregnancy. *Br. J. Obstet. Gynaecol.* **82**, 100.

ROBINSON H. P. & FLEMING J. E. E. (1975) A critical evaluation of sonar crown–rump length measurements. *Br. J. Obstet. Gynaecol.* **82**, 702.

CHAPTER 4

Real-time ultrasound in the second and third trimesters of pregnancy

M. J. Bennett

As has been seen from previous chapters, ultrasonic examination of the pregnant patient by means of real-time equipment is a relatively simple and quick procedure. The fact that a thorough knowledge of the physics of ultrasound is not required for the efficient use of this equipment is of great importance to the practising obstetrician. Equally important is the fact that the majority of real-time machines have very few controls and thus efficient use of this equipment is quite easily learned.

It is important to appreciate that real-time transducers allow a rapid 'search' of the pregnant uterus to be made and, from this initial examination, the precise areas to be examined in more detail can be readily identified.

THE BASIC QUESTIONS

There are a number of basic questions which need to be answered when considering the ultrasonic examination of any patient who is thought to be pregnant. The questions are as follows:

1 Is the patient pregnant?
2 If so, what is the gestational age?
3 How many fetuses are present?
4 What proof is there of fetal viability?
5 Where is the placenta situated?

Is the patient pregnant?

It is well known that ultrasonic examination of the uterus can readily identify the presence of a gestation sac within a few weeks of conception. As has been seen in Chapter 3 the diagnosis of early pregnancy by means of real-time equipment can be made, but there are certain requirements. The first of these is that the patient must have a full urinary bladder in order that the uterus can be adequately identified. Given this proviso it must be appreciated that the gestation sac becomes visible when real-time apparatus is used something like a week to two weeks after it would normally be visible when a static scanner is used. This means that, although a pregnancy can be diagnosed at $5–5\frac{1}{2}$ weeks of gestational age by means of a static scanner, it will only be as readily identified by means of real-time equipment at around 6–7 weeks. This is because the resolution of the currently available real-time transducers is not as good as that of most static scanners. Nevertheless, the diagnosis of pregnancy can be positively made before the second missed menstrual period and at about the same time as a urinary test for human chorionic gonadotrophin can be expected to be positive.

The diagnosis of a continuing pregnancy depends upon the demonstration of a live fetus within the gestation sac. With a static scanner, fetal viability can be demonstrated from the 7th week of pregnancy onwards and once again something like a week or two must be added to this when real-time equipment is used. Robinson has shown that a gestational sac with a volume greater than 2.5 ml must always contain a fetus. The absence of fetal echoes in a gestation sac of greater volume permits the ultrasonic diagnosis of an anembryonic pregnancy to be made.

In the presence of signs and symptoms of pregnancy, the absence of a gestational sac within the uterus should not be taken as positive proof that the patient is not pregnant. In the first instance, the sac may be so small that it cannot be identified with real-time apparatus. In the second, implantation may not have occurred within the uterine cavity and an ectopic pregnancy may be present. It is therefore wise to give the patient the benefit of the doubt and to re-evaluate the situation a week or two later, provided the clinical situation does not indicate a different course of action. An extra-uterine pregnancy is an exceedingly difficult diagnosis to make with ultrasonic equipment at the best of times and is even more difficult when real-time equipment alone is used.

What is the gestational age?

The question of gestational ageing is one of the most fundamental to obstetricians. For the last ten years ultrasound has provided the obstetrician with the best method of assessing gestational age and this is likely to remain the case. It is best to discuss the assessment under two separate headings.

First trimester

As has been adequately demonstrated in Chapter 3, the ultrasonic measurement of the crown–rump length provides the most accurate method of assessing the duration of gestation. Adam *et al* (1979) have shown not only that the measurement of this parameter by means of real-time equipment is possible, but that the correlation between this form of equipment and the more conventional static scanner is an extraordinarily good one. Our unit has also shown that the correlation coefficient is better that $r = 0.9$. In order to achieve an accurate measurement of crown–rump length, the ultrasonic equipment must have not only freeze-frame facilities, but also a set of omni-directional calipers.

Once the fetus is identifiable on the screen, a crown–rump length can be measured. However, if the pregnancy has entered the last few weeks of the first trimester the crown–rump length becomes more difficult to measure because of the naturally curved shape of the fetus at this stage. Nevertheless, crown–rump measurements are vastly superior to any other form of measurement that can be achieved in the first trimester and should therefore always be preferred.

Second and third trimesters

Measurement of the fetal biparietal diameter (BPD) during the second and third trimesters of pregnancy has been used for many years as the ultrasonic parameter of gestational age. The initial work of Campbell (1968) is well known to all obstetricians and is as valid today as when first published. The fetal head becomes ultrasonically visible in virtually every instance from the 13th week onwards — although it is sometimes visible and can be measured during the 12th week of pregnancy. The ability of real-time equipment to allow a rapid search of the pregnant uterus to be made greatly facilitates identification of the fetal head.

In order that the gestational age can be reliably inferred from the BPD, close attention to the technique of measurement is vital. The lie and presentation of the fetus are easily determined throughout the second and third trimesters. Occasionally, problems are encountered in locating the head when it is deeply engaged in the pelvis during the third trimester but, by a systematic examination, its position can usually be ascertained. The fetal head remains the most easily definable structure throughout both these trimesters with a

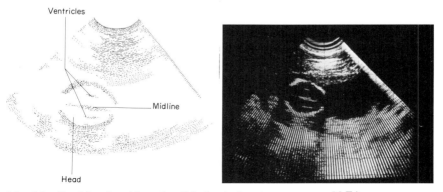

Fig. 4.1 Fetal head at 15 weeks. (Mechanical sector scanner — N.E.)

strong midline echo seen in transverse sections. The origin of this midline echo is not clear but the cerebral falx is thought to be the most likely site. The technique used in this ultrasound unit was described by Campbell in 1968 and is as follows:

First, a longitudinal scan is made to determine the angle of the fetal head to the vertical axis (the angle of asynclytism). The probe is then rotated through 90° and inclined to the previously measured angle of asynclytism. This section should give a true transverse view of the fetal head which appears as an ovoid with a midline echo bisecting it. If the midline echo is not apparent, the longitudinal scan should be repeated, as either the angle of asynclytism has been incorrectly measured or the fetus has moved. Once the transverse section of the fetal head has been obtained, the picture is best 'frozen' by means of the freeze-frame facility. This ensures that any subsequent movement will not impede measurement of the BPD. The ultrasonic callipers are then placed in such a way that they measure the distance between the maximum convexities of the parietal bones. If these callipers are single dots then they ought to be placed on the leading edges of the near and far parietal bones. If they are horizontal lines, they should be placed at right angles across the leading edges of the two parietal bones. Some real-time apparatus allows a single trans-ducer to be selected and an A-scan picture to be displayed on the side of the screen. A system with this facility permits the exact placement of the callipers to be checked and thereby a more accurate reading to be obtained. After a single measurement has been taken, subsequent measurements are made both caudal and cephalad to this first transverse scan to establish the widest transcoronal diameter. Measurements may only be made if the midline echo is still midway between the two parietal bones. In prac-tice, the true transverse plane giving maximum biparietal skull width will show a discontinuous midline as a result of the presence of the third ventri-cal. The stronger, continuous midline echo is seen in a plane at a more cephalad level and does not represent the largest diameter of the skull. When the fetus is presenting by the breech, fetal head movements result-ing from maternal respiratory effort often make measurement very diffi-cult. Accuracy is, however, quite possible if the real-time equipment has a freeze-frame facility and the patient is asked to hold her breath for a short time. Care should be taken in interpretation of the BPD measure-ment in breech presentation since the head will often be slightly deformed and the BPD measurement slightly less than would be expected for a fetus of that age. In fact, this is only apparent in the third trimester of pregnancy. In a controlled study performed in this unit, measurements were obtained from over 300 patients by two separate operators, one of whom was using a real-time linear array system and the other a conventional static scanner. The correlation coefficient of the two sets of readings was $r = 0.998$ (Fig. 4.2). During the course of this study, one of the major difficulties of the

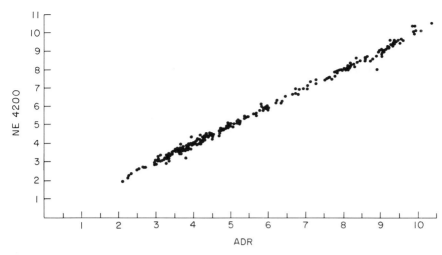

Fig. 4.2 Comparison of BPD measurements between a conventional scanner (NE 4200) and a linear array scanner (ADR).

large transducer associated with a linear array system became apparent: occasionally the combination of the shape of the maternal abdomen, the position of the fetal head and the size of the transducer did not allow an accurate BPD reading to be obtained. In this study it was found that 15% of BPD measurements were not regarded as accurate and were therefore discarded. Sector scanners (mechanical or electronic) perform much better in this respect since the small area of contact of the transducer is very similar to that of a conventional scanner transducer; the number of occasions on which a BPD cannot be accurately measured with these transducers is less than 1%.

It can therefore be seen that accurate BPD measurements with real-time equipment are very readily obtained and preliminary data from Robinson and Adam suggest that these measurements can be obtained in a third of the time used to obtain similar measurements with a static scanner.

A single BPD measurement will predict gestational age to within ± 1 week provided that it is obtained before the 24th week of pregnancy. It is widely accepted that the estimation of gestational age from such a single measurement obtained after 32 weeks of gestation is not sufficiently accurate to be of any clinical value. Attention should also be paid to the calibration velocity used to determine the measurement. The initial work of Campbell was made using a velocity of 1600 m/sec. but others have used different velocities. This means that, if an already published graph is to be used as the reference for BPD measurements, it must have been obtained using the same velocity as the machine upon which the measurements are to be made. Failure to appreciate this point results in errors which may be of clinical significance.

How many fetuses are present?

The diagnosis of a multiple pregnancy can only be made when fetuses can readily be identified and counted. It is well known that a significant number of pregnancies which result in the birth of a single fetus have been found shortly after conception to have more than one gestation sac in the uterus. The incidence of this occurrence is not known, but some authorities estimate

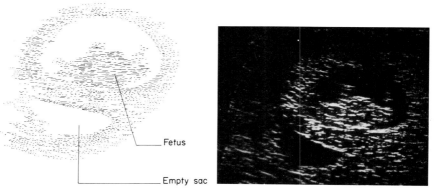

Fig. 4.3   An example of two gestational sacs with the upper one containing a fetus and a lower empty one.

that it is as high as 20% of all pregnancies. Fig. 4.3 shows quite clearly the presence of a single fetus with a small empty sac below it. Two weeks after this picture was obtained, a repeat ultrasonic examination failed to reveal any evidence of the second sac. It is quite obvious from this and many similar

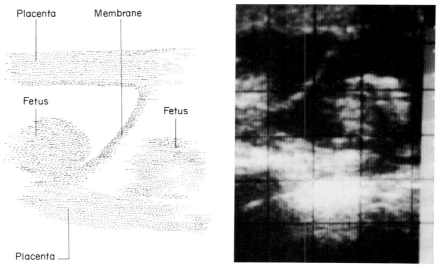

Fig. 4.4   Twin fetuses at 14 weeks demonstrating two separate sacs. (ADR 5.0 MHz transducer.)

illustrations that a diagnosis of multiple pregnancy on the basis of the number of gestation sacs could have been made some weeks earlier but would have been an erroneous one. It is therefore of paramount importance to identify individual fetuses before a diagnosis of multiple pregnancy can be made.

With a gestational age of more than 8 weeks a multiple pregnancy should never be missed on ultrasonic examination, be it with real-time or static equipment. During the second trimester, the presence of two individual fetal heads can readily be shown and the transducer aligned in such a way as to display both heads on the same section (Fig. 4.4). Nevertheless, difficulties are encountered in the diagnosis of multiple pregnancy, particularly when there are three or more fetuses present in the uterus. It can, then, be concluded that the earlier the diagnosis is made the more accurate the count is likely to be. The increased incidence of multiple pregnancy following stimulation of ovulation should make the ultrasonographer very wary of making a diagnosis after a cursory examination. It is impossible to over-emphasize the value of seeing patients who have conceived as a result of the induction of ovulation both soon after conception and repeatedly if the correct diagnosis is to be made.

What proof is there of fetal viability?

One of the greatest advantages of real-time ultrasound as far as the patient is concerned is the ability to diagnose fetal life. Embryologically the fetal heart starts to beat within 4 weeks of conception. Fetal heart movement can be shown by means of static scanners using a TM mode by the 7th week of gestational age. Using real-time apparatus, the fetal heart can invariably be seen to beat at the 9th gestational week and occasionally a week earlier. The real-time facility allows not only the fetal heart to be identified but also actual fetal movements to be seen and, of equal importance, shown to the patient.

There is no pathological situation which can mimic the movements made by a live fetus and therefore whether a fetus is live or not should never be in doubt when real-time facilities are used after the 8th week. The same is true of the movements occurring within the fetal heart and, provided the duration of pregnancy is greater than 8 or 9 weeks, the diagnosis of the presence of a live fetus can always be made. The diagnosis of multiple pregnancy can therefore confidently be made if more than one live fetus is seen.

Where is the placenta situated?

It is only after the 12th week of pregnancy that the placenta becomes an ultrasonically discernible separate entity. Prior to this, it is sometimes possible to predict which part of the gestation sac will ultimately become the placenta but such a prediction has no clinical relevance. The placenta appears from the beginning of the second trimester onwards as a soft grey shadow occupying a portion of the uterine wall. The chorionic plate, separating the placental tissue from the amniotic fluid, shows up as a firm white line and as such helps to differentiate the placenta from an area of thick myometrium. From an ultrasonic point of view, however, identification of the placenta is only one aspect of localization. The other is of course the accurate delineation of the limits of the placenta. Should the placenta be seen to lie in the fundus of the uterus, then — even during the early part of the second trimester — a confident diagnosis which excludes placenta praevia can be made. The reverse is, however, a trap into which the unwary often fall.

Prior to the 32nd week of pregnancy there is, for practical purposes, no lower segment. It is therefore impossible, by definition, to make a diagnosis of a placenta praevia. It is however quite possible to diagnose a 'low lying placenta' and, in these circumstances, a repeat examination after the 32nd week of pregnancy is vital.

REAL-TIME ULTRASOUND IN THE MANAGEMENT OF ABNORMAL PREGNANCY STATES DURING THE FIRST TRIMESTER

The most common abnormalities occurring in the first trimester of pregnancy include: threatened, incomplete or complete abortion, anembryonic pregnancy, missed abortion and, more rarely, hydatidiform mole and ectopic pregnancy.

In each case the patient is likely to present with one or more of the following symptoms: signs of early pregnancy, vaginal bleeding to a greater or lesser degree and, sometimes, lower abdominal pain. It is thus difficult for the clinician to make a definitive diagnosis and the additional help of an ultrasonic examination will often confirm the diagnosis for him.

Ultrasonic findings

Anembryonic pregnancy

This is a pregnancy in which trophoblast develops but no embryo forms. As has been previously stated, the first ultrasonic evidence of a pregnancy is a small, clearly defined sac with a trans-sonic central area. A week or so later fetal echoes can be identified if the pregnancy is a normal one. Robinson has defined an anembryonic pregnancy as being one in which the volume of the gestation sac is greater than 2.5 ml and in which there are no fetal echoes. The problem with this diagnosis is that the gestation sac is seldom circular and thus volumetric calculation becomes exceedingly difficult. Obviously when a large gestation sac is seen and there are no fetal echoes, a confident diagnosis of anembryonic pregnancy can be made. Conversely, when a small sac is seen which contains no fetal echoes, it is best to give the benefit of the doubt to the pregnancy and to re-examine the patient a week or even two later. If no fetus is then evident, the diagnosis of an anembryonic pregnancy can be made and the clinician has to decide whether he wishes to surgically evacuate the uterus or to allow nature to take its course.

Abortion

One of the commonest problems facing the clinician is the patient who presents with some vaginal bleeding after a short episode of amenorrhoea. It should be evident from the foregoing that an ultrasonic examination will, in most instances, diagnose whether or not the patient has an intra-uterine pregnancy and, provided the pregnancy is far enough advanced, whether or not the fetus is live. In the past, the management of patients threatening to abort relied very heavily upon a combination of bed rest and repeated urinary pregnancy tests. With real-time ultrasonic facilities, the management is now much more rational and once a diagnosis has been made the appropriate management can be instituted. In a retrospective study of over 1000 patients who presented in this ultrasound department with a clinical diagnosis of threatened abortion, it was found that if a live fetus was identified despite the bleeding then only 8% of the patients subsequently aborted. Once again if a definitive diagnosis of a non-continuing pregnancy is made, the clinician is left to decide whether or not the uterus requires surgical evacuation of its contents. With real-time ultrasound, if a live fetus can be demonstrated, the patient cannot only be reassured but can be shown the evidence for this reassurance, i.e. a live fetus. Those who have managed patients in this manner will know the tremendous relief and gratitude displayed by patients under these circumstances.

The diagnosis of an incomplete abortion can equally readily be made on a single ultrasonic examination. Retained products of conception within the cavity of the uterus have a very characteristic appearance and should neither be missed nor mistaken for anything else.

The diagnosis of an ectopic pregnancy is not a diagnosis that ultrasound can be reliably depended upon to confirm. In the patient who presents with signs and symptoms of pregnancy, vaginal bleeding and lower abdominal pain, the absence of any intra-uterine evidence of pregnancy should make the clinician consider the possibility of an ectopic pregnancy more strongly. Very occasionally, a gestation sac is seen quite clearly separate from the uterus and, under these circumstances, laparatomy will usually confirm the ultrasonic suspicion of an ectopic pregnancy. The presence of an intra-uterine gestation sac will usually exclude the diagnosis of an extra-uterine pregnancy, but there have recently been a number of isolated reports in the literature in which such an appearance was seen despite the presence of an ectopic pregnancy. It is therefore unwise ever to make a negative diagnosis on the basis of an ultrasonic examination.

Hydatidiform mole

This uncommon condition has very typical ultrasonic features. To the in-experienced it seems as though the entire uterus is filled with placental tissue and no evidence of either a fetus or amniotic fluid can be found. Before making such a diagnosis, however, one must be careful to examine the whole uterus both longitudinally from one side to the other as well as transversely from the top to the bottom. A single section taken through a laterally implanted placenta will produce a picture indistinguishable from that of a hydatidiform mole and it is only on complete scanning in both longitudinal and transverse planes that it can be identified as placenta.

With the very high levels of circulating hCG associated with this condition, one can almost always see theca lutein cysts in one or both ovaries. These are readily seen as extra-uterine, echo-free, multilocular masses. However, the diagnosis of hydatidiform mole may be made even if these theca lutein cysts are not seen.

Vaginal termination of pregnancy

In situations where termination of pregnancy is permitted, it is important for the gynaecologist to know whether or not it is safe to terminate the pregnancy vaginally. Notwithstanding the foregoing section on gestational age, there are two simple points which the gynaecologist would do well to remember, i.e. the fetal head and the placenta — both of which can only easily be identified (particularly by the ultrasonically inexperienced) once the second trimester has begun (Fig. 4.5). It is therefore fairly safe to say that, if by means

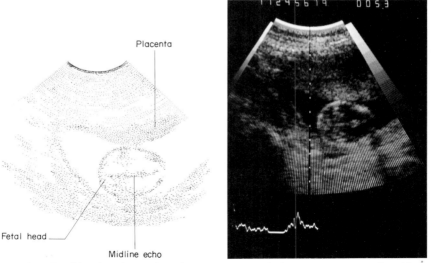

Fig. 4.5   Fetal head and anterior placenta. (Mechanical sector scanner—Combison 100.)

of an ultrasonic examination (real-time or compound scanning) either the fetal head or the placenta can be clearly identified, then it is probably no longer safe to terminate the pregnancy vaginally. This is quite obviously a rule of thumb but one which we have found a very useful one to pass on to junior staff.

ULTRASONIC EVALUATION OF FETAL GROWTH

Growth and maturation, although very closely related, are not inseparable. For example, the large fetus of the diabetic mother is, in some respects, functionally less mature than a fetus of equal size and age born to a non-diabetic mother. Another example is the small growth-retarded baby whose functional maturity is often considerably in advance of that of an equal sized baby which is appropriately grown for its age. Thus it can be seen that gestational age, growth and functional maturity are in fact separate entities which may progress at different rates. It is therefore unwise to infer the existence of one from an assessment of another.

In assessing fetal growth, a mandatory prerequisite is knowledge of the gestational age. At the beginning of this chapter it was stressed that the earlier such an assessment was made the more accurate it would be. For the purposes of this section, it will be assumed that gestational age is known — for without it growth rates cannot be evaluated.

The simplest method of measuring growth is by means of serial BPD measurements. Unfortunately this is not the best method in view of the brain-sparing ability of the fetus, i.e. where intra-uterine nutrition is sub-optimal the fetal brain is spared proportionately more than the rest of the body. This results in the classic build of a 'small-for-dates' baby — the small, long

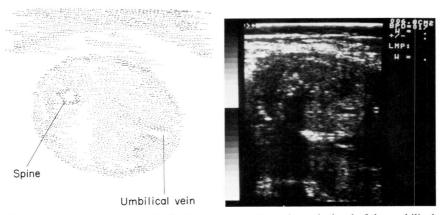

Fig. 4.6 Transverse section of a fetal abdomen at 24 weeks at the level of the umbilical vein. (Roche Superscan 50.)

thin body with a disproportionately large head (even if this is smaller than expected for the baby's gestational age).

It is therefore appropriate to use an additional parameter and there are many to choose from in the literature. Since the pathologist relates the weight of the liver to the weight of the brain as an index of the degree of malnutrition, it would make sense for the obstetrician to attempt to do the same. An ultrasonically determined parameter such as the diameter of the upper abdomen or the lower thorax is unquestionably the easiest to obtain, but equally these provide the least information. Campbell and Wilkin (1975) describe the use of a circumferential measurement of the fetal abdomen at the level of the umbilical vein and relate it to the circumference of the fetal head in the occipito-frontal plain. By this technique they claimed to be able to diagnose 87% of growth-retarded fetuses when measurements were made between 32 and 34 weeks.

The inability to compound a picture obtained with real-time apparatus sometimes leads to the failure to display the complete fetal trunk or head circumference. Nevertheless, we have found that, when an acceptable picture can be obtained, clinically applicable measurements can be made (Fig. 4.6).

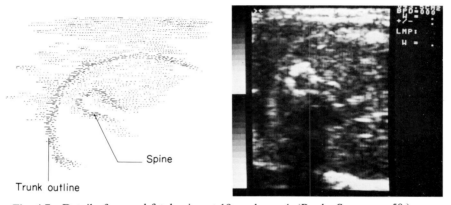

Fig. 4.7 Detail of normal fetal spine at 19 weeks, × 4. (Roche Superscan 50.)

In general, measurements of this sort should not be taken at intervals of less than two weeks in order to reduce the error inherent in the method. There can be no doubt that routine ultrasonic measurements of the above sort performed at 32–34 weeks, even with real-time apparatus, will diagnose a much higher proportion of growth-retarded fetuses than will the clinician.

ULTRASONIC DETECTION OF FETAL ABNORMALITIES

Ultrasound is unable to detect the majority of the structural abnormalities of the fetus. Nevertheless certain abnormalities have been identified; the most

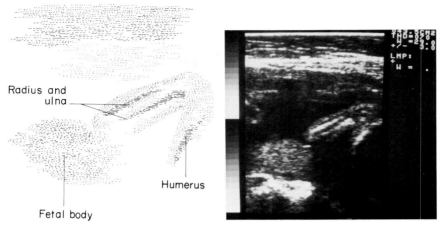

Fig. 4.8   Both forearm bones in a fetus of 26 weeks. (Roche Superscan 50.)

easy of these being anencephaly. This diagnosis can and should always be made prior to the 18th week of pregnancy by virtue of the absence of the cephalic pole. Although other defects of the neural tube, including spina bifida and hydrocephalus, have been identified by real-time apparatus, the relatively poor resolution of this apparatus at present makes the diagnosis of these abnormalities almost impossible on routine examination. Diagnoses of such rare conditions as exomphalos, renal agenesis and duodenal atresia have been reported, but, again, none but the most highly skilled are likely to recognize such conditions on routine examination.

The potential for the diagnosis of fetal cardiac malformations is discussed in Chapter 6.

REFERENCES

ADAM A. H., ROBINSON H. P. & DUNLOP C. (1979) *Br. J. Obstet. Gynaecol.* **86**, 521.
CAMPBELL S. (1968) *J. Obstet. Gynaecol. Br. Commonw.* **75**, 568.
CAMPBELL S. & WILKIN D. (1975) *Br. J. Obstet. Gynaecol.* **82**, 689.

CHAPTER 5

The use of ultrasound in fetoscopy

G. R. Devore & J. C. Hobbins

Fetoscopy, a term which describes the direct visualization of the fetus in its intra-uterine environment, has become a useful diagnostic tool of the perinatologist and geneticist. Prior to the use of fetoscopy, the main vehicle of genetic sampling was amniocentesis. Although amniocentesis allows one to screen for a number of chromosome anomalies, X-linked diseases, and more than 82 biochemical disorders and congenital malformations, over 90% of fetal cells in the amniotic fluid are dead or dying and the fluid itself does not express all of the metabolic functions of the fetus (Henry *et al* 1978, Sandstrom & Milunsky 1977, Rhine 1976, Simpson & Martin 1976).

Fetoscopy allows one to sample fetal cells directly either by biopsy or by blood sampling and has been useful in the diagnosis and evaluation of a number of genetic disorders, many of which were incompletely evaluated with amniocentesis alone (Table 5.1) (Hobbins & Mahoney 1977, Burton & Nadler 1977, Levine *et al* 1974, Mahoney *et al* 1977, Mahoney & Hobbins 1977, Mahoney & Hobbins in Press, Rodeck & Campbell 1978, Benzie 1977, Laurence *et al* 1974, Firshein *et al* in Press, Newburger *et al* in Press, Alter *et al* 1976).

Initially, researchers examined fetuses prior to elective termination of pregnancy using a pediatric cystoscope 5–6 mm in diameter. Unfortunately, most pregnancies sampled were associated with interruption because of the size of the instrument used (Golbus 1977, Phillips 1977). Currently most fetoscopists are using a non-flexible, solid rod endoscope (Fig. 5.1, Hobbins & Mahoney 1976). The image is carried by a solid self-focussing lens surrounded by fibres which transmit light into the uterine cavity. This lens and fibre system measures 1.7 mm in diameter by 15 cm in length. When inserted into the uterus, it is housed in a 2.2 mm diameter cannula. The endoscope has a depth of focus of about 2 cm, an angle of visualization of 70° and permits a view of 2–4 cm² at one time with a × 25 magnification. If the endoscope is brought close to the surface of the tissue to be visualized, higher magnification is achieved. Most fetoscopies have been done with a percutaneous insertion of the endoscope using only local anaesthesia at the insertion

Table 5.1　Some genetic disorders whose study is facilitated by fetoscopy.

Genetic disease	Fetoscopic evaluation	Reference
Sickle cell anaemia	Fetal blood	Hobbins & Mahoney 1977, Alter *et al* 1976, Alter & Nathan 1978
B thalassaemia major	Fetal blood	Hobbins & Mahoney 1977, Alter *et al* 1976, Alter & Nathan 1978
Duchenne's muscular dystrophy	Fetal blood	Mahoney *et al* 1977
Chondroectodermal dysplasia (Ellis–van Creveld Syndrome)	Fetal visualization	Mahoney & Hobbins 1977
Other skeletal dysplasias　Polydactyly　Syndactyly　Abnormal thumbs　Hypoplastic radii　Facial clefts　Single limb amelia	Fetal visualization	Mahoney & Hobbins, in Press, Benzie 1977, Laurence *et al* 1974
Meningomyelocele, spina bifida	Fetal visualization	Mahoney & Hobbins, in Press, Benzie 1977, Laurence *et al* 1974
Classic haemophilia	Fetal blood	Firshein *et al*, in Press
Chronic granulomatous disease	Fetal blood	Newburger *et al*, in Press
Fetal skin defect (Harlequin Syndrome)	Fetal scalp biopsy	Hobbins & Mahoney 1976

site. The pregnancies have been 15–20 weeks' gestation and intra-uterine viewing time has been 10–50 minutes. Before 15 weeks the uterus is too small easily to enter with the current method of endoscopy. Because of the limited visual field, ultrasound is invaluable in the localization of fetal tissues for visualization and/or sampling purposes.

Fetoscopy has now advanced to the point where it is used as a diagnostic tool in women desiring to maintain their pregnancy if, after the appropriate test, a genetic disorder in the fetus can be excluded. As of October 1978, we have studied 98 patients: the fetuses of 8 patients were examined by direct visualization, while in 90 patients an attempt was made to sample fetal blood by fetoscopy or placental aspiration. In those in whom we were unable to obtain blood by direct visualization, placental aspiration was performed. The complications have been minimal with only 4 patients undergoing spontaneous abortion after the procedure (less than the 10–20% reported in the literature for placental aspiration; see also Table 5.2, Alter *et al* 1976, Kan *et al* 1974).

Ultrasound has been used by some investigators to localize the placenta 24 hours prior to the procedure (Benzie & Pirani 1977). Our perinatal unit

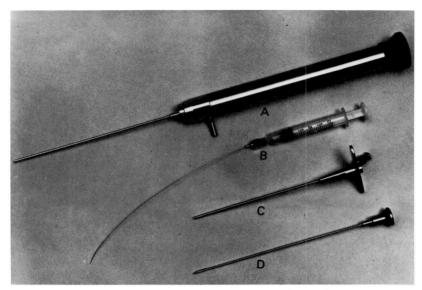

Fig. 5.1 Instruments used during fetoscopy. A Needlescope[R], B 26-gauge needle used for aspiration of blood, C Cannula with Y piece through which the needle is inserted, D Trochar.

Table 5.2 Comparison of methods.

	Fetoscopy	Placental aspiration
Patients studied	84	14
visualization alone	8	—
attempted fetal blood sampling	76	14
Patients who chose termination based on prenatal diagnosis	16	2
Patients who chose termination without diagnostic data	2	1
Pregnancies continued	66	11
stillborn	1 (1.5%)	0
spontaneous abortion	3 (4%)	1 (9%)
premature delivery	6 (9%)	0
vaginal bleeding	0	0
intermittent leakage of amniotic fluid	2 (3%)	0
mild transient abdominal pain	7 (11%)	7 (64%)
fever or post-operative infection	1 (1.5%)	0
term delivery	45 (68%)	10 (91%)
undelivered	11 (17%)	0

uses ultrasound prior to and during the entire procedure. The following pages describe the use of ultrasound in the patient undergoing fetoscopy for 1 fetal blood sampling, 2 visualization of fetal parts and 3 tissue biopsy.

Equipment

 B-mode ultrasound
 Real-time ultrasound
 Y-shaped cannula
 1.7 mm endoscope with light source
 26-gauge needle
 Biopsy forceps
 Appropriate sterile precautions.

FETAL BLOOD SAMPLING

An initial B-mode contact scan is performed using a higher frequency transducer of 3.5 or 5 MHz firstly to locate the site of attachment of the placenta to the uterine wall and its dimensions and, secondly, to determine the position and lie of the fetus. A pocket of amniotic fluid is chosen which will afford a safe entry into the amniotic cavity. If a posterior placenta is noted, then a point on the abdominal wall is entered which lies over the fetal small parts (Fig. 5.2). If an anterior placenta is noted, a search is made for a placenta-free window through which the fetoscope can be inserted (Fig. 5.3). In our previously reported description of blood sampling (Hobbins & Mahoney 1976), the use of A-mode ultrasound was an integral part of ultrasound evaluation. The tip of the Y-shaped cannula housing the endoscope, when passed through a transducer on the abdominal wall, emits an echo on the oscilloscope of the A-mode ultrasound which is separate from the other intra-abdominal echoes. This allows the operator to determine exactly where the endoscope is within the intra-uterine cavity (Fig. 5.4). Currently we no longer use A-mode ultrasound, but use real-time ultrasound. When using real-time ultrasound the contact solution is Betadine (*Napp*) and the abdomen is widely draped. Once the cannula and endoscope are inserted into the uterine cavity, one can determine the level of the tip by directional manipulation of the real-time transducer. For example, if the transducer array is perpendicular to the cannula, one will see a solid circumscribed echo on the screen. By changing the angle of inclination one can follow the cannula to its tip (Fig. 5.5). If one desires to view the cannula in its entire length, then the array should be placed parallel to the direction of the cannula. With this approach, however, the slightest movement laterally will displace the image from the screen (Fig. 5.6). As the placenta is approached, the fetoscopist can then visualize the placental vessels with the fetoscope. Once a suitable vessel is located, it is pierced with a 26-gauge needle inserted into and through the side of

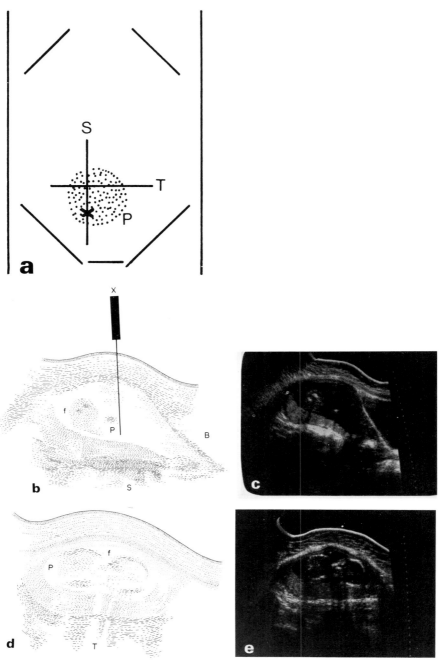

Fig. 5.2 Fetoscopic approach with a posterior placenta. S sagittal scan to the right of the umbilicus, T transverse scan. P placenta, X insertion site of the Needle-scope[R], B bladder, f fetus. The transverse scan demonstrates an area without fetal parts which is safe for the fetoscopic approach.

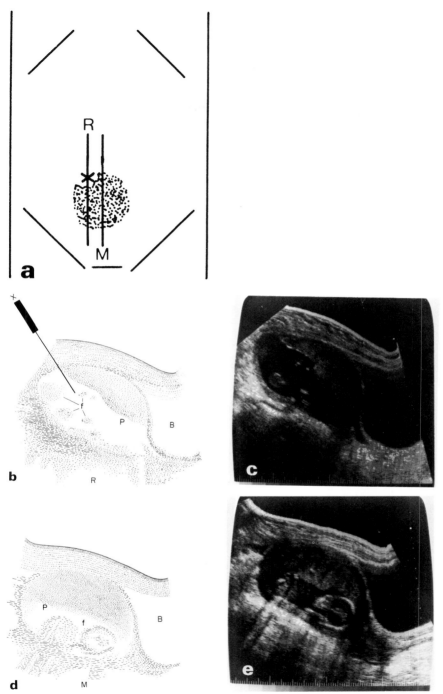

Fig. 5.3 Fetoscopic approach with an anterior placenta. R sagittal scan to the right of the midline, M midline sagittal scan, X insertion site of the Needlescope[R]. P placenta, B bladder, f fetus. The scan through the midline demonstrates the anterior placenta and fetus without a placenta window. The right sagittal scan demonstrates a placenta-free window through which the fetal surface of the placenta can be approached for sampling.

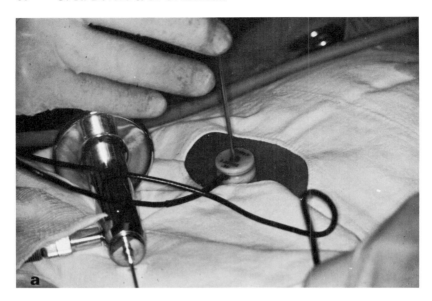

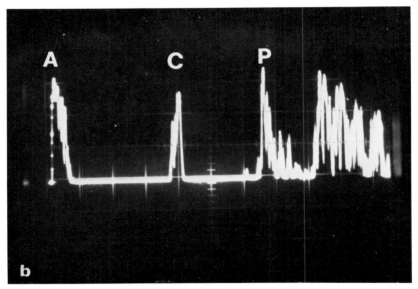

Fig. 5.4   Use of A-mode ultrasound. **a** demonstrates the transducer of the abdominal wall through which the cannula and trochar are passed. **b** is the A-mode display illustrating the abdominal wall A, the tip of the cannula C and the placenta P.

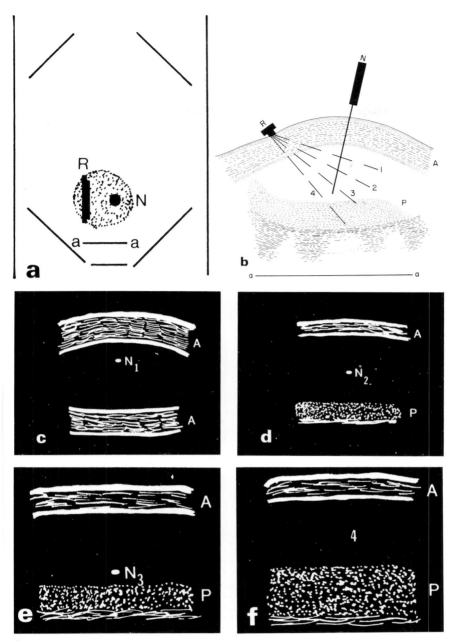

Fig. 5.5 Use of real-time ultrasound to locate the depth of the fetoscope in the intra-uterine cavity. R real-time transducer, N Needlescope[R]. P placenta, a–a area of the abdominal cavity represented, A anterior abdominal wall. **a** illustrates the position of the real-time transducer on the abdominal wall when scanning perpendicular to the Needlescope[R], **b** illustrates the relationship of the transducer when scanning perpendicular to the Needlescope[R]. 1–4 are the areas scanned as illustrated in **c–f**, which show what is seen on the real-time display. N_1–N_3 are bright spots seen on the screen at each level representing the Needlescope shaft. When one loses the image of the Needlescope shaft, that is the depth of the tip.

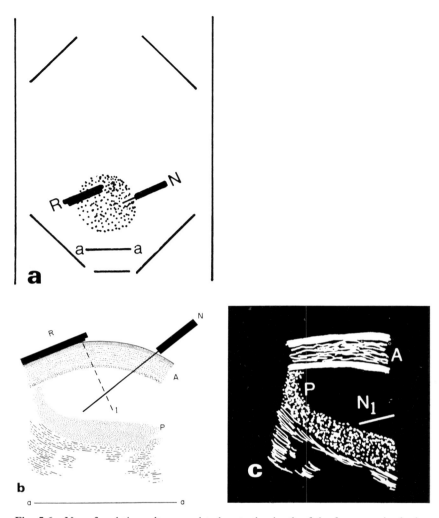

Fig. 5.6 Use of real-time ultrasound to locate the depth of the fetoscope in the intra-uterine cavity. R   real-time transducer, N   Needlescope[R], a–a   area of the abdominal cavity represented, P   placenta, A   anterior abdominal wall. **a** illustrates the position of the real-time transducer when scanning parallel to the Needlescope[R]. **b** is the cross-sectional area through a–a representing the relationship of R to N. **c** illustrates what is seen on the real-time display. The Needlescope[R] shaft (N_1) appears as a bright line.

the Y-shaped cannula. When one aspirates fetal blood, it is important to remember that aspiration is not intravascular (as in an adult) but is extravascular. The fetal blood is aspirated as it is extruded from the punctured vessel into the adjacent amniotic fluid (Fig. 5.7). Approximately 1 cc of blood and amniotic fluid is removed. In some cases it has been possible to obtain a

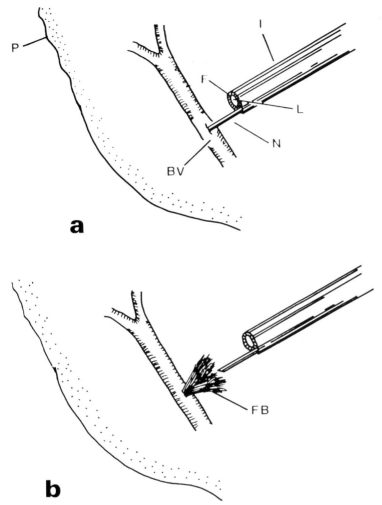

Fig. 5.7 Fetal blood sampling. P placenta, BV blood vessel, F fibre-optic light source, L lens, I introducer cannula, FB fetal blood. **a** illustrates the 26-gauge needle within the fetal blood vessel. **b** illustrates fetal blood exuding from the vessel and the tip of the needle aspirating amniotic fluid and fetal blood.

sample from the vessel, but this is difficult because of its small diameter. It has been noted that bleeding from the puncture site stops almost immediately.

Placental aspiration

If one is unable to obtain fetal blood because of an anterior placenta and either unsuccessful or unattempted fetoscopy, placental aspiration is indicated. The technique is relatively simple. The placenta is localized and the margins clearly delineated with grey scale. Using a high frequency needle aspiration transducer with a small hole, or by reference to the displayed video picture, a 20-gauge spinal needle is directed to the location of the tip just inside the chorionic plate, where 0.1–0.3 ml of blood is aspirated into a heparinized syringe. Many small samples are then obtained at different levels within the placenta, and a sample is also obtained from the amniotic fluid adjacent to the punctured placenta. These samples are generally mixed with an appreciable percentage of maternal blood, but one must obtain at least 5% fetal cells for haemoglobin studies. The maternal blood obtained is undoubtedly from the intravillous space, and the fetal blood must be coming from traumatized fetal cotyledons and/or vessels (Fig. 5.8).

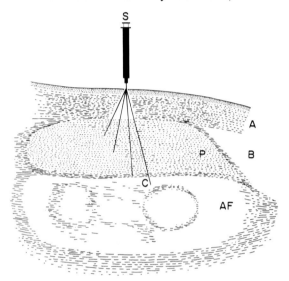

Fig. 5.8 Placental Aspiration. S   syringe and needle, P   placenta, B   bladder, A   anterior abdominal wall, AF   amniotic fluid, C   chorionic plate. This illustrates the various depths in the placental tissue from which aspiration is performed.

VISUALIZATION OF FETAL PARTS

As with fetal blood sampling, an initial B-mode scan is performed to locate the site of attachment of the placenta to the uterine wall and its dimensions, the position and lie of the fetus, the biparietal diameter for gestational age calculation, and a pocket of amniotic fluid which will afford a safe entry into the amniotic cavity. Real-time ultrasound is used, as in fetal blood sampling, to examine the area of the fetus to be visualized. The limbs, for example, are evaluated if one is looking for major limb defects (Ellis–van Creveld Syndrome or split-hand deformity), or the spine and skull in patients where neural tube defects are suspected (Fig. 5.9). Once this is done, a placenta-free area is selected over the area to be examined by the fetoscope. During

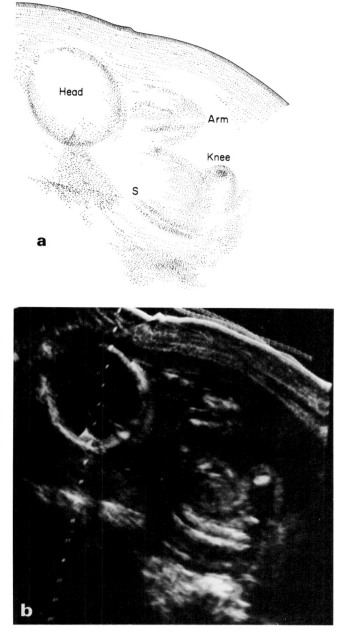

Fig. 5.9   Scan of fetal extremities. **a** is an illustration of the scan, **b** demonstrating fetal small parts, spine, and head.

the fetoscopic procedure, real-time ultrasound is very useful to relocate parts of the fetus and direct the fetoscopist to them. The fetus is usually very active and its movements can be helpful in bringing areas like hands or feet into view. Fetal movements can also be frustrating and at times fetal sedation with diazepam is useful. If the area to be examined is not in an optimal position, one can usually manipulate the fetus to the desired position for feto-

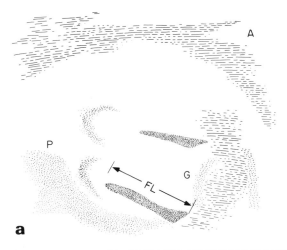

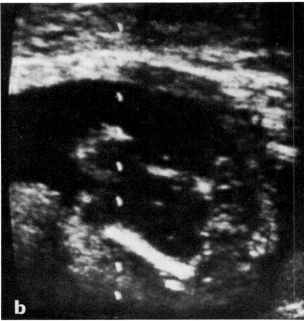

Fig. 5.10   Measurement of femur length. **b** illustrates what is seen in the scan **a** P   placenta, FL   femur length, G   genital area, A   abdominal wall.

scopy by placing the mother on her side, in the knee–chest position or, using ultrasound, by gently guiding the fetus into the proper area for evaluation. Because the visual field is limited, one usually cannot visualize the entire fetus during a single procedure; thus a degree of selectivity is required. This underlines the importance of proper ultrasound evaluation prior to fetoscopic examination. In one patient with Ellis–van Creveld Syndrome, for example, we were able to measure the length of fetal extremities (Fig. 5.10) and to identify a postaxial sixth digit, which confirmed the diagnosis of limb shortening that was suspected using ultrasound (Fig. 5.11).

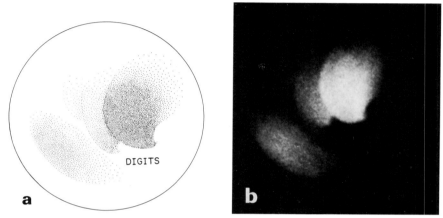

Fig. 5.11 Visualization of fetal digits. **a** illustrates what is seen in **b** through the fetoscope. Three digits are visualized.

TISSUE BIOPSY

Using the same procedure as for fetal blood sampling, an initial B-mode ultrasound examination surveys the fetus and determines the position of the placenta. Once a placenta-free window is noted and the fetal skull located, the cannula with the endoscope is inserted through the abdominal wall. Using real-time ultrasound the position and depth of placement of the cannula tip can be ascertained as in fetal blood sampling. Once the fetal skull is approached, endoscopic evaluation of the area is carried out. The proper area for biopsy is determined by noting hair in all four quadrants of the visual field. When the desired area over the fetal scalp has been located, the endoscope is removed and biopsy forceps are inserted and proximity to the scalp gauged using real-time ultrasound. Once the biopsy forceps are in place, tissue biopsy is performed (Fig. 5.12). If fetal movements occur from the time the endoscope is removed and the biopsy forceps inserted, the procedure is begun again. The advantages of fetal scalp sampling are that 1 the head is protected by the calvaria, 2 it rarely moves, 3 it bleeds little, and 4 it also provides hair on which to perform biochemical analysis (Fig. 5.13).

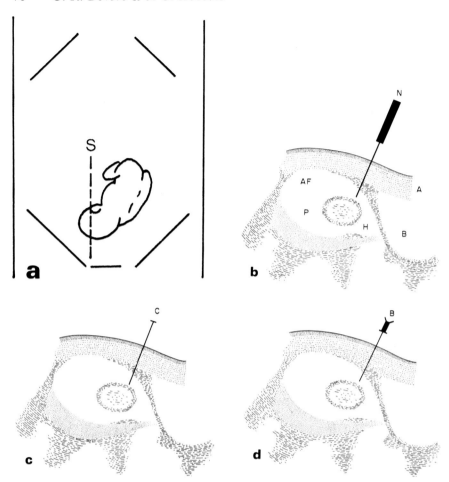

Fig. 5.12 Fetal scalp tissue biopsy. S   sagittal scan, AF   amniotic fluid, P   placenta,
H   fetal head, B   bladder, A   anterior abdominal wall, N   Needlescope[R], C   introducer cannula, B   biopsy forceps. **a** illustrates the relationship of the sagittal scan to
the fetus and abdominal wall, **b** demonstrates the Needlescope in visualizing the fetal
scalp, **c** illustrates removal of the Needlescope with the introducer cannula in place and
d demonstrates the biopsy forceps in place.

CONCLUSION

Fetoscopy has allowed the perinatologist and geneticist access to the fetal
compartment which provides unlimited diagnostic potential. Ultrasound is
a component of pre-fetoscopic evaluation and is essential during the procedure to appreciate spatial relationships. Without the use of both contact
and real-time ultrasound, it is our feeling that the safety and efficacy of fetoscopy would be greatly jeopardized.

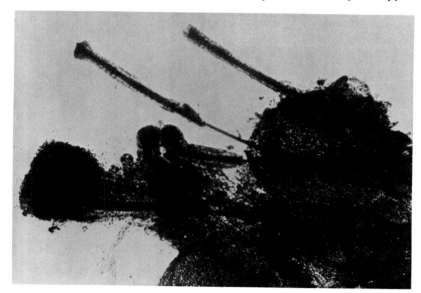

Fig. 5.13 Fetal scalp tissue.

REFERENCES

ALTER B. P., MODELL M. D., FAIRWEATHER M. D. *et al* (1976) Prenatal diagnosis of hemoglobinopathies: A review of 15 cases. *N. Engl. J. Med.* **295,** 1437.

ALTER B. P. & NATHAN D. G. (1978) Antenatal diagnosis of haemotological disorders. *Clin. Hematol.* **7,** 195.

BENZIE R. J. (1977) Fetoscopy. In *Embryology and Pathogenesis and Prenatal Diagnosis,* eds., D. Bergoma and R. B. Lowry. Birth Defects: Original Article Series **13,** (3D), 181.

BENZIE R. J. & PIRANI B. B. (1977) Fetoscopy and anterior placentas (letter). *N. Engl. J. Med.* **296,** 573.

BURTON B. K. & NADLER H. L. (1977) Prenatal diagnosis of biochemical defects. *Contemp. Obstet. Gynecol.* 10L39.

FIRSHEIN S. I., HOYER L. W., LAZAREHCH J. *et al.* Prenatal diagnosis of classic hemophilia. In Press.

GOLBUS M. S. (1977) Fetal blood sampling in continuing pregnancy. Read in Fetoscopy Seminar, 3rd International Congress on Gynecologic Endoscopy, San Francisco.

HENRY G. P., PEAKMAN D. C. & ROBINSON A. (1978) Prenatal genetic diagnosis: nine years experience. *Ob/gyn Surv.* **33,** 569.

HOBBINS J. C. & MAHONEY M. J. (1976) Fetoscopy and fetal blood sampling: the present state of the method. *Clin. Obstet. Gynecol.* **19,** 341.

HOBBINS J. C. & MAHONEY M. J. (1977) Fetoscopy in continuing pregnancies. *Am. J. Obstet. Gynecol.* **129,** 440.

KAN Y. W., VALENTI C., GUIDOTTI R. *et al* (1974) Fetal blood sampling *in utero. Lancet* i, 79.

LAURENCE K. M., PEARSON J. F., PROSSER R. *et al* (1974) Fetoscopy followed by live birth. *Lancet* i, 1120.

LEVINE M. D., McNEIL D. E., KABACK M. M. *et al* (1974) Second trimester fetoscopy

and fetal blood sampling: current limitations and problems. *Am. J. Obstet. Gynecol.*
120, 937.

MAHONEY M. J., HASELTINE F. P., HOBBINS J. C. *et al* (1977) Prenatal diagnosis of
Duchenne's muscular dystrophy. *N. Engl. J. Med.* **297**, 968.

MAHONEY M. J. & HOBBINS J. C. (1977) Prenatal diagnosis of chondroectodermal dys-
plasia (Ellis–van Creveld Syndrome) with fetoscopy and ultrasound. *N. Engl. J.
Med.* **297**, 258.

MAHONEY M. J. & HOBBINS J. C. Fetoscopy in the prenatal diagnosis of skeletal abnormalities. In Press.

NEWBURGER P. E., COHEN H. J., ROTHCHILD *et al* The prenatal diagnosis of chronic
granulomatous disease: superoxide generation by fetal leukocytes. In Press.

PHILLIPS J. M. (1977) Fetoscopy: direct visualization and sampling of the fetus, an over-
view. *Acta Endoscp. Radiocinematogr.* **8**, 55.

RHINE S. A. (1976) Prenatal genetic diagnosis and metabolic disorders. *Clin. Obstet.
Gyn.* **19**, 855.

RODECK C. H. & CAMPBELL S. (1978) Early prenatal diagnosis of neural tube defects
by ultrasound-guided fetoscopy. *Lancet* i, 1128.

SANDSTROM M. M. & MILUNSKY A. (1977) Prenatal genetic diagnosis. *Am. Fam. Phys.*
15, 121.

SIMPSON J. C. & MARTIN, A. O. (1976) Prenatal diagnosis of cytogenic disorders. *Clin.
Obstet. Gyn.* **19**, 841.

CHAPTER 6

Real-time assessment of fetal and neonatal cardiac dynamics

J. W. Wladimiroff, R. Vosters & W. Vletter

The arrest of the umbilical circulation and the increase of pulmonary flow on ventilation of the lungs immediately following delivery will result in marked circulatory changes in the newborn: the foramen ovale closes, the ductus arteriosus constricts. It is clear that these changes must have a significant effect on left and right ventricular function. Real-time two-dimensional ultrasound devices have led to the possibility of more detailed studies of cardiac structures in relation to their movement.

The purpose of this chapter is to discuss the assessment — before and after birth — of:

1 Left and right ventricular size;
2 intraventricular septal motion;
3 left and right ventricular ejection time.

The ultrasonic system

A real-time linear array ultrasonic scanner was used with a dynamic focussing system. This focussing system, with a phased array of twelve elements, resulted in a lateral resolution of about 2 mm over the entire field of view. The fundamental frequency of the array was 3.12 MHz. Using a multi-element transducer consisting of 51 elements, a rectangular image with 40 lines was built up. Video processing techniques were applied to compose a high line-density ultrasonic image on a television monitor.

Two single beam transducers were used for antenatal and neonatal M-mode recording. The frequency was 2.25 and 5.0 MHz, the diameter 13 and 6 mm.

Recording techniques

In our antenatal studies, a B-mode cross-section of the fetal chest showing spine and heart is first obtained. Next, a single beam transducer is positioned at an angle of 45° to the antero–posterior diameter of the fetal chest in

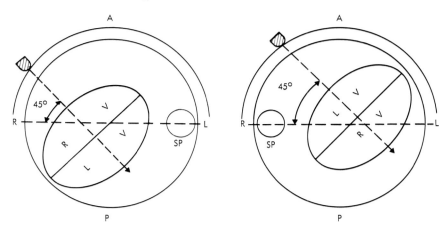

Fig. 6.1 Cross-section of fetal chest showing spine (SP) and heart. The single beam transducer is positioned at an angle of 45° to the antero-posterior diameter of the fetal chest. A left lateral position of the fetal spine will result in an approach from the right ventricle; a right lateral position of the fetal spine will result in an approach from the left ventricle.

order to be approximately at right angles to the intraventricular septum (Fig. 6.1). A left lateral position of the fetal spine will result in an approach from the right ventricle (Fig. 6.1a), whilst a right lateral position of the fetal spine will result in an approach from the left ventricle (Fig. 6.1b).

The final step is a so-called 'M-mode cardiac scan', which will lead

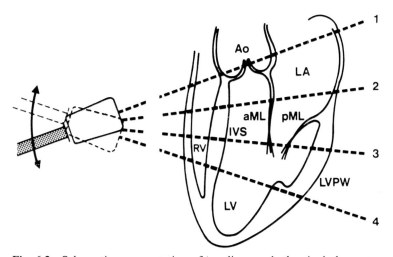

Fig. 6.2 Schematic representation of 'cardiac scan': the single beam transducer has to move from plane 1, via plane 2 to plane 3 which is the correct plane representing the left and right ventricle (LV and RV), the intraventricular septum (IVS) and anterior and posterior mitral valve leaflet (aML and pML). Ao aortic root, LA left atrium, LVPW left ventricular posterior wall.

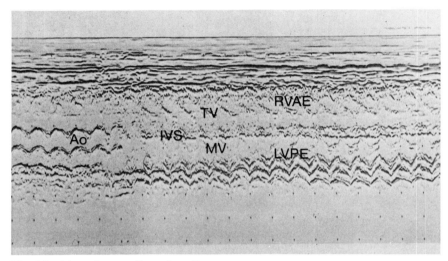

Fig. 6.3 M-mode recording of cardiac scan.
LVPE left ventricular posterior endocard, RVAE right ventricular anterior endocard, TV tricuspid valve, MV mitral valve. Note that aortic root (Ao) and intraventricular septum (IVS) are situated at the same level of the recording.

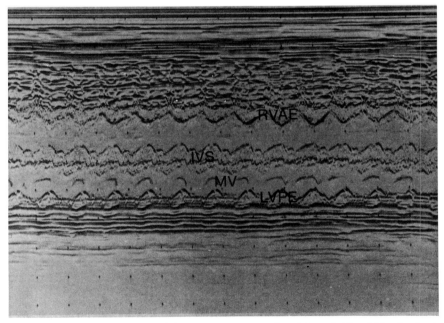

Fig. 6.4 M-mode recording of the correct cross-section (plane 3, Fig. 6.2) of a fetal
heart at 37 weeks gestation.

us to the correct plane of investigation. Fig. 6.2 gives the sequence of scans involved. The recording is started at right angles to the aortic root, which is characterized by two nearly parallel moving echoes (plane 1). The transducer is subsequently moved down towards the apex of the heart (plane 2), ultimately showing the correct scanning plane consisting of the left and right ventricular wall, the intraventricular septum, and the anterior and posterior mitral valve leaflet (plane 3). During this procedure, the aortic root and intraventricular septum should be appearing at the same level of the M-mode tracing. This confirms the correct position of the transducer, which is at right angles to the intraventricular septum (Fig. 6.3). In our neonatal studies, only a single beam transducer was used as the position of the heart was known.

Fig. 6.4 demonstrates an M-mode recording of the cross-section just described of a fetal heart at 37 weeks of gestation, showing the endocard of the left ventricular posterior wall, the mitral valve leaflet, the intraventricular septum and endocardium of the right ventricular wall. Fig. 6.5 shows the same cross-section in a two-day-old infant.

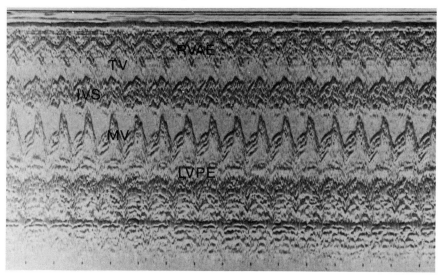

Fig. 6.5   The same cross-section in a two-day-old infant.

Patients and methods

In the first part of our study we looked at 11 antenatal patients. Pregnancies were normal; pregnancy duration varied from 34 to 41 weeks. In the second part of our study, we focussed our attention on the period around delivery. In 6 normal pregnancies, M-mode recordings were made:

  within 24 hours of delivery;
  within 10 minutes following delivery;
  4 hours following delivery;
  1, 2 and 3 days following delivery.

In each M-mode recording the following measurements were performed:

left and right ventricular diameter in the end-diastolic position in mm;
left to right ventricular ratio;
end-diastolic and end-systolic position of the intraventricular septum;
left and right ventricular ejection time in milliseconds, determined by the
time interval between opening and closing of pulmonary and aortic valve;
heart rate.

The reproducibility of each of the ventricular diameters and ejection time
measurements was assessed from ten M-mode recordings of the same patient
performed on the same day. This was done in a pregnancy of 38 weeks and

Table 6.1 Reproducibility of measurements based on ten consecutive
recordings of one patient.

	Antenatal		Postnatal	
	$\bar{X}$	$\pm$ 1 s.d.	$\bar{X}$	$\pm$ 1 s.d.
LV (ED) (mm)	14.1	0.74	17.0	0.67
RV (ED) (mm)	14.5	0.71	9.7	0.48
LVET (msec)	194	10.1	190	10.4
RVET (msec)	190	10.0	185	10.1

a one-day-old infant (Table 6.1). It was decided to measure each of the parameters five times and subsequently calculate the mean value.

Results

Table 6.2 gives the left and right ventricular dimension, left to right ventricular ratio, left and right ventricular ejection time and heart rate of the 11 fetuses
in the first part of our study. Right ventricular diameter varied from 13.8
to 19.6 mm; left ventricular diameter varied from 13.7 to 18.8 mm. Left to
right ventricular ratio varied from 0.92 to 1.05. Right ventricular ejection
time ranged from 172 to 202 msec. and left ventricular ejection time varied
from 174 to 201 msec. Fetal heart rate varied from 125 to 150 b.p.m.

Fig. 6.6 demonstrates the relationship between left (open circles) and right
ventricular diameter (closed circles) and birth weight. A positive correlation
seems likely; however, more data are needed.

The data derived from the second part of this study will be presented
in the next figure.

Fig. 6.7a gives the left and right ventricular end-diastolic dimension (open
and closed circles respectively), the left to right ventricular ratio, the left and
right ventricular ejection time (open and closed circles) and heart rate, within
24 hours of delivery (I), immediately following delivery (II), four hours (III),
one day (IV) and two days following delivery (V).

Table 6.2   Measurements taken from antenatal patients of 34–41 weeks.

Patient	L.V. dimen-sion (mm)	R.V. dimen-sion (mm)	L.V./R.V. ratio	L.V. ejection time (msec)	R.V. ejection time (msec)	Fetal heart rate (b.p.m.)
1	16.3	16.7	0.99	184	180	135
2	15.6	14.9	1.05	176	176	145
3	14.0	13.8	1.01	188	190	130
4	18.8	18.5	1.02	174	172	150
5	18.0	17.9	1.0	187	185	140
6	16.2	17.4	0.93	201	202	130
7	17.3	16.9	1.02	194	197	125
8	13.7	14.0	0.97	178	180	140
9	16.1	17.5	0.92	174	178	145
10	18.4	19.6	0.94	184	181	140
11	14.5	14.5	1.0	188	183	135

This patient was delivered at 38 weeks. Immediately following delivery there was a moderate increase in left ventricular diameter from 14.6 to 17.6 mm accompanied by a marked reduction in right ventricular diameter from 15.2 to 10.2 mm. The ratio went up from 0.95 to 1.7. Both right and left ventricular diameters stay virtually unaltered in the first two days following delivery. The left and right ventricular ejection time showed a very slight difference and varied from 190 to 204 msec. A slowing down in heart rate from 130 to 110 b.p.m. is associated with a slight rise in left and right ventricular ejection time.

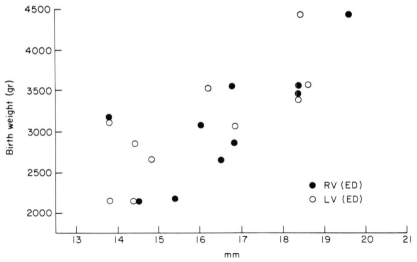

Fig. 6.6   Relationship between left (open circles) and right ventricular diameter (closed circles) and birthweight.

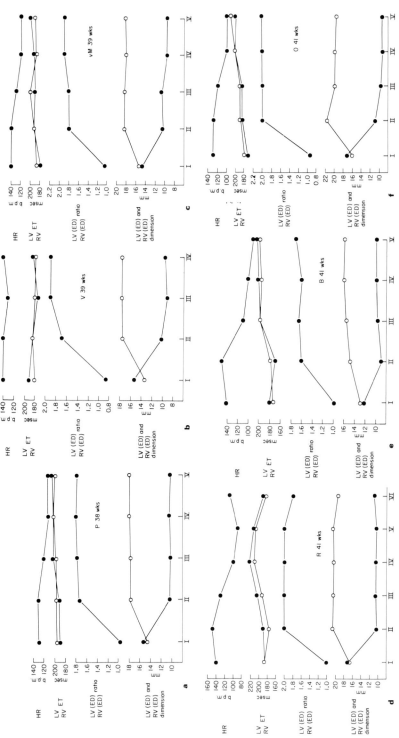

Figs. 6.7 Left and right ventricular end-diastolic dimension (open and closed circles respectively), left to right ventricular ratio, left and right ventricular ejection time (open and closed circles) and heart rate within 24 hours of delivery (I), immediately following delivery (II), 4 hours (III), one day (IV) and two days following delivery (V).

Fig. 6.7b demonstrates a patient of 41 weeks. Left ventricular diameter increased from 13.4 to 17.4 mm, right ventricular diameter reduced from 15.6 to 10.2 mm. In contrast to the left ventricular diameter, the reduction in right ventricular diameter continued until the first day post-partum. The ratio went up from 0.9 to 1.7 to 1.9. The left and right ventricular ejection times varied from 176 to 190 msec. Fig. 6.7c represents a patient of 39 weeks, demonstrating a similar pattern of moderate increase in left ventricular diameter and marked reduction in right ventricular diameter, the ratio going up from 1.0 to 1.8 immediately after the delivery. A slight further rise in ratio on day 1 was determined by slight further reduction in right ventricular diameter. The left and right ventricular ejection time varied from 180 to 200 msec. Fetal heart rate slowed down from 140 to 120 b.p.m.

Fig. 6.7d demonstrates a patient who was followed-up to 3 days post-partum. The left ventricular diameter increased from 16.5 to 20.0 mm, and the right ventricular diameter went down from 16.5 to 10.2 mm. The ratio doubled from 1.0 to 2.0, only to return to a slightly lower level of 1.8 on day 3. An increase in left and right ventricular ejection time is associated with a reduction in fetal heart rate and vice versa.

The fifth patient (Fig. 6.7e), also at 41 weeks, demonstrates a pattern very similar to that of the previous patient. An enlargement of the left and a reduction of the right end-diastolic ventricular diameter immediately following delivery, also expressed by the increase in ratio from 1.0 to 1.6. The further follow-up is characterized by a very small increase in left and right ventricular diameter. Again, a negative relationship can be observed between the left

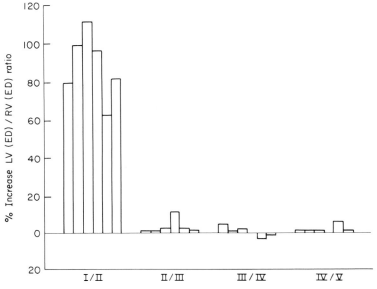

Fig. 6.8 Change in left to right ventricular ratio immediately following delivery (I/II), 4 hours (II/III), one day (III/IV) and two days (IV/V) following delivery.

and right ventricular ejection time, varying from 170 to 206 msec., and the heart rate varying from 150 to 90 b.p.m.

The findings from the last patient are shown in Fig. 6.7f. A marked increase in left and a marked decrease in right ventricular diameter immediately following delivery can be observed. The ratio went up from 0.85 to 1.9. The left and right ventricular ejection time is again inversely related to the heart rate.

The diagram in Fig. 6.8 underlines once more the impressive increase in left to right ventricular ratio immediately following delivery in the six patients just presented. The percentage increase varied from 62.5 to 112%. Four hours later and on days 1 and 2, no significant change in ratio can be observed.

Finally, the results of the study on intraventricular septal movement were as follows: In the antenatal period, the pattern of intraventricular septal movement varied substantially amongst the patients studied. Patterns from normal to paradoxal were observed. An example of paradoxal intraventricular septal movement is shown in Fig. 6.9. In the neonatal period, the septal movement was always normal, that is the septum was moving towards the posterior wall of the left ventricle during systole.

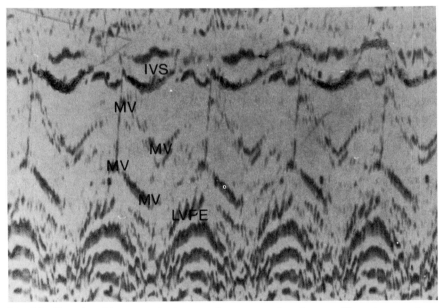

Fig. 6.9 Paradoxal intraventricular septal movement in a fetus at 38 weeks gestation. LVPE left ventricular posterior endocardium, MV mitral valve, IVS intraventricular septum.

Conclusion

1 Ventricular size demonstrates a left to right ratio varying from 0.85–1.05 before birth to 1.4–2.0 during the first 3 days following delivery.

2   The increase in ventricular left to right ratio following delivery is determined more by reduction in right ventricular size than by an increase in left ventricular size. It is realized though, that only one of the three ventricular dimensions has been studied.

3   The major changes in ventricular size seemed to occur immediately following delivery. At that time the percentage of increase in ventricular left to right ratio varied from 62.5 to 112%.

4   The pattern of intraventricular septal movement during pregnancy varied from normal to paradoxal. This is probably determined by the degree of right ventricular overload present at the time. Similar findings were shown by Hobbins *et al* (1978). A closer antenatal study of the time relationship between intraventricular septal movement and ventricular wall movement is needed. Patterns were normal in the neonatal study.

5   Left and right ventricular ejection times varied from 170 to 220 msec.; a relationship to heart rate seems likely.

Finally, simultaneous recording of mechanical and electric cardiac activity will undoubtedly provide us with a deeper insight into the changes of cardiac dynamics around birth.

REFERENCE

HOBBINS J. C., KLEINMAN C., CREIGHTON D. (1978) Fetal Echocardiography: Indirect evaluation of *in utero* fetal flow patterns. *Proc. Soc. Gynecol. Invest.* 25th Annual Meeting, Atlanta, p. 48.

CHAPTER 7

Reproducibility of real-time ultrasound fetal measurements

D. J. Little

With the increasing availability of real-time ultrasound equipment, members of the obstetric team are able to perform ultrasound examinations in the wards and clinics. This is in sharp contrast to static or B-scanning where large, expensive machines are located in separate departments and require highly trained operators if they are to achieve satisfactory results. One of the major determinants of the relative roles of static and real-time scanning is the relative accuracy of their measurements; this is reflected by their reproducibility. A second consideration is how appropriate are normal data obtained by static scanning in the interpretation of real-time measurements.

Real-time ultrasound is not merely an alternative to static scanning, its ease and speed of use offers the potential to screen the obstetric population for gestational age, i.e. prediction of the estimated date of delivery (EDD), and for fetal growth. The following discussion considers the accuracy and reproducibility of real-time measurements and compares these with the results found in clinical practice.

REPRODUCIBILITY OF REAL-TIME ULTRASOUND MEASUREMENTS

The reproducibility of measurements of the biparietal diameter (BPD) and circumference of the fetal head and abdomen was studied in 20 patients using both a static and a real-time scanner. The reproducibility was expressed as the mean standard deviation of three measurements per patient.

Static scan measurements were made using a Diasonograph N.E. 4200 (Nuclear Enterprises, Edinburgh). The BPD was measured by the combined A-B-scan technique (Campbell 1968). The head circumference was measured at the level of the third ventricle (Campbell 1976) and the abdominal circumference at the level of the umbilical vein (Campbell & Wilkin 1975) within the fetal liver.

Real-time measurements were made with an ADR linear array scanner

(ADR Corp., Arizona) with a 3.5 MHz transducer. The ADR was equipped with a video monitor, electronic calipers (Kretz-Technic UK) and a calibrated polaroid system. Circumferences were measured on the polaroid photographs with a map measurer. Head measurements were made without a preliminary longitudinal scan, the head was scanned transversely and the transducer angled until a strong midline echo was displayed bisecting the head. The BPD and circumference were then measured at this angle.

Two-thirds of the group were first examined on the static scanner and one-third on the real-time scanner. Once the BPD, head and abdominal circumferences had been measured, the patient walked to a separate room and a second series of measurements was made on the alternative machine. The time interval between the first and second measurement of each variable on the same machine ranged from 20 minutes to 3 hours. All BPD measurements were obtained 'blind'. The circumference measurements were made after the polaroid photographs had been randomly mixed. Each polaroid photograph was coded to allow the patient to be identified after the measurement had been made.

REPRODUCIBILITY OF BIPARIETAL DIAMETER MEASUREMENTS

Twenty volunteers were selected from the women attending the Obstetric Ultrasound Unit at King's College Hospital. The gestational ages ranged from 17 to 40 weeks, 16 were vertex presentation and 4 presented by the breech.

The mean standard deviation of three measurements was 0.52 mm for static scan and 0.83 mm for real-time scanning. This difference is statistically significant ($t = P < 0.02$), although in clinical practice a difference of this small size is not important. The difference between the first and second measurement was compared to the difference between the first and third measurement for each patient, i.e. those measurements closest and furthest apart in time. There was no significant difference, confirming the independence of the measurements. Comparison of the reproducibility of measurement of the 10 smallest and 10 largest heads revealed no difference. Lunt and Chard (1974) have suggested that reproducibility is better for heads in the BPD range of 59–83 mm, but this series does not confirm this.

The published studies of the comparative reproducibility of static and real-time measurement of the BPD are summarized in Table 7.1. Cooperberg and co-workers (1976) measured the BPD from polaroid photographs for both techniques, while Docker and Settatree (1977) used similar techniques to the present study (see later for a fuller discussion). It is interesting that the reproducibility of real-time measurements was similar in all three studies, that is with mean standard deviations of approximately 1 mm. In comparison, static scan reproducibility shows much greater variation. The published

Table 7.1   Reported mean standard deviations for static + real-time measurement of the BPD. Note that the real-time reproducibility ± 1 mm for all series.

	Static scan (mm)	Real-time (mm)	*P*
Little	0.52	0.83	< 0.02
Cooperberg *et al* 1976	0.91 BS	0.77	
	0.69 GS		
Docker & Settatree 1977	1. 1.13	1.09	< 0.05
	2. 1.77	1.18	< 0.001

S Significant difference, BS Bistable scan, GS Grey scale scan

mean standard deviations vary from 0.25 mm (Campbell 1970) to 2.03 mm (Davison *et al* 1973), which suggests that operator variation is less significant for real-time scanning than static scanning. Docker and Settatree's data illustrate the point: the real-time scan reproducibility was about 1 mm for both workers whose experience was widely different, whereas a clinically significant difference in the static scan reproducibility was shown, i.e. 1.13 mm for the experienced operator versus 1.77 mm for the less experienced operator.

In using BPD measurements to assign a gestational age, the confidence limits depend on the accuracy of the individual measurement plus the biologic range of BPDs for a given gestational age. As described above, two standard deviations for real-time measurement of the BPD is ± 2 mm. This corresponds to ± 4 days between 14 and 28 weeks menstrual age, i.e. at a time when EDD predictions are made. Using Campbell and Newman's (1971) normogram for BPD versus menstrual age and Campbell's (1969) mean standard deviation of 0.25 mm for measurement in early pregnancy, the 95% confidence limits for real-time prediction of the EDD should be ± 10 days. It is important to note that, in the hands of most workers, static scanning does not offer a clinically significant improvement in the accuracy of measurement of the BPD and hence of predicting the EDD.

The agreement between real-time and static scan measurements

Results

When the mean BPD measured by real-time scanning is plotted against that measured by static scanning a close correlation is clearly present (Fig. 7.1). The BPD measured by real-time scanning is significantly smaller than that measured by static scanning (Table 7.2). When the series is divided into the 10 smallest and 10 largest heads it is apparent that the difference arises in the measurement the largest heads. This indicates that, in making predictions of the EDD from real-time measurements of BPD before 24 weeks (i.e. small heads), data derived from static scanning studies may be used.

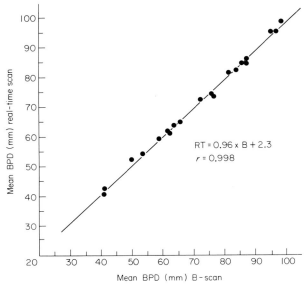

Fig. 7.1   Comparison of mean BPD measured by real-time and by static scanning.

Discussion

Static scan normal data were obtained by measuring from the anterior surface of the anterior parietal bone (= outer) to the anterior surface of the posterior parietal bone (= inner). This is the most precise measurement as it is based on the leading edges of the skull bone echo complexes. The visualization of the posterior surfaces of the parietal bones depends on the decay of the signal and is affected by the processing of the signal and the setting of the gain controls. Caliper measurements on unmoulded heads suggested that, by assigning 1600 m/sec. as the speed of sound when measuring outer to inner, the best approximation to the anatomical BPD is obtained (Willocks *et al* 1964). The average speed of sound in human tissues is 1540 m/sec. The 4% increase in the result entailed in using 1600 m/sec. effectively allows for the thickness of the posterior parietal bone when measuring outer to inner. Campbell used static scan measurements outer to inner at 1600 m/sec. in compiling his normogram (Campbell & Newman 1971) and this should be the

Table 7.2   Mean BPD measured by real-time + static scanning. The agreement is closest for the ten smallest heads.

	B-scan	Real-time	*P*
20	72.2	71.6	0.001
Smallest 10	57.3	57.5	NS
Largest 10	87.1	85.6	0.001

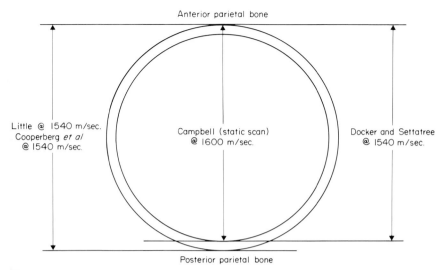

Anterior parietal bone

Little @ 1540 m/sec.
Cooperberg *et al*
@ 1540 m/sec.

Campbell (static scan)
@ 1600 m/sec.

Docker and Settatree
@ 1540 m/sec.

Posterior parietal bone

Fig. 7.2   Values used in BPD measurement.

preferred real-time technique. None of the studies has used this technique (Fig. 7.2).

In the present study the measurement was made outer to outer at 1540 m/sec. as personal experience suggested that it was easier to apply horizontal bar calipers to a moving convex surface than to a concave (i.e. inner) surface cut by the caliper line. This is not the case with spot calipers or freeze-frame images and studies are under way to assess these systems. Cooperberg *et al* measured outer to outer on polaroid photographs at 1540 m/sec. and found a close correlation between the two techniques. Measuring outer to outer at 1540 m/sec. is equivalent to outer to inner at 1600 m/sec. $\pm$ the error due to the variation in the apparent thickness of the posterior parietal. The magnitude of this error remains to be determined. Docker and Settatree measured outer to inner at 1540 m/sec. and observed a good correlation between the real-time and static scan measurements. They suggested that the agreement would be improved by adding 1 mm to the real-time measurements. Recalibration of their equipment to 1600 m/sec. would add 4% to the real-time measurements throughout the range and could not account for this observation.

Despite these difficulties all the reports agree that the use of normal data obtained by static scanning is not associated with clinically significant errors.

CLINICAL EXPERIENCE OF REAL-TIME SCANNING IN ASSIGNING THE GESTATIONAL AGE

Women attending the antenatal clinic for booking at King's College Hospital are routinely examined with a linear array real-time scanner (ADR + Diagnostic Sonar System 85 scanners). The records of the first 610 patients were analysed. In 319 of them the EDD was determined by a certain menstrual history or a static scan measurement of the BPD before 24 weeks. Campbell (1976) has shown that the latter is significantly more accurate than a certain menstrual history in predicting the onset of spontaneous labour resulting in the delivery of a mature fetus. This prediction was compared to the EDD predicted from real-time measurement of the crown–rump length or of the BPD (Table 7.3, Robinson 1973).

Table 7.3   Correlation between the EDD predicted by a certain menstrual history or a static scan BPD measurement before 24 weeks gestational age and that predicted by a single real-time measurement of the crown–rump length or BPD at the booking visit.

	n	Mean difference in predictions	s.d. $\times$ 1	r
Crown–rump length before 14 weeks	91	$+3.4$ days	5.4 days	0.85
Biparietal diameter				
13–17 weeks	166	$+0.18$	4.9	0.93
17–21 weeks	62	$+0.21$	6.2	

The 95% confidence limits, i.e. ± 2 standard deviation for the real-time predictions, were very close to the ± 10 days predicted by the reproducibility data. The mean error in the real-time prediction was virtually zero for the BPD-based predictions thus supporting the use of static scan-derived normal data. Crown–rump-based predictions were significantly later than the dates/static scan EDD; the most likely reason for this is the difficulty in defining the fetal poles in polaroid photographs of still real-time images. The use of freeze-frame will allow immediate on-screen measurement and better selection of the optimal image for measurement.

Clinical implications

Real-time measurement of the BPD offers a similar level of accuracy as static scanning in predicting the EDD in the hands of average workers. The 95% confidence limits of ± 10 days are wider than the ± 7 days derived from the data of Campbell and Newman (1971) for static scan BPD measurement in early pregnancy and the ± 5 days reported by Robinson for static-scan crown–rump measurements. One way of increasing the precision of real-time predictions is by taking two measurements before 24 weeks as has been shown for static scanning. Campbell (1976) reported that when a single BPD measurement was used to assign the EDD, 84% of patients delivered within ± 14 days of the predicted date. Only patients delivering mature fetuses after a spontaneous onset of labour were considered. By using two BPD measure-

Table 7.4 Reasons for doubt about EDD prediction based on the menstrual history in 488 patients.

Uncertain recall of the date of the LMP	19.6%
Irregular menstrual cycle (greater than 8 days)	2.9%
Oral contraceptive use within two months of conception	9.8%
Bleeding in early pregnancy	1.6%
Multiple factors	4.7%
	38.6%

ments to assign the EDD, Varma (1973) observed that 91% delivered within ± 9 days of the predicted date.

Of women attending King's College Hospital, 40% had some reason to doubt the EDD predicted by the menstrual history. The reasons are outlined in Table 7.4.

Although it is logical to select these 40% with doubtful dates for ultrasound scanning in early pregnancy, in practice only total screening at booking will ensure that all these patients are examined. It would be sensible to reexamine these women before 24 weeks and use the two measurements in assigning the EDD. This could be confined to those with serious doubt about their menstrual history and those in whom the menstrual age and real-time-assigned gestational age differ by more than 7 days. Although more accurate prediction of the EDD is desirable, in some ways it offers diminishing returns in assisting patient management. The critical question in managing abnormal pregnancies is not the precise gestational age but the functional maturity of the fetal organ systems, especially the lungs. The latter is subject to wide biologic variation and is not simply a function of the gestational age. It is also influenced by pathologic states, e.g. acceleration of lung maturation in fetal growth retardation and slowing in diabetes.

Increased precision may be important in interpreting biochemical and other data dependent on the fetal age, e.g. amniotic fluid AFP levels in prenatal diagnosis and abdominal circumference measurements in following fetal growth.

REPRODUCIBILITY OF CIRCUMFERENCE MEASUREMENTS

Two patients were excluded from the analysis of the abdominal circumference results as the fetal outlines in the polaroid photographs of real-time scanning were not sufficiently well defined to be measured. Fetal movement greatly enhances the perception of the fetal outlines in real-time scanning. This is a useful aid if the image is measured immediately from the polaroid photograph and conversely makes measurement after a time interval more difficult.

Head circumference

The mean standard deviation for three measurements of 20 patients was 0.33 cm for static scan and 0.57 cm for real-time scanning. This difference is statistically significant ($t = P < 0.02$). There was no variation of the reproducibility with head size. Linear regression confirms the close agreement between the static and real-time scan measurements ($r = 0.998$). The mean circumferences measured by the two techniques did not differ significantly.

Abdominal circumference

Abdominal circumference measurements were compared in 21 patients. As shown in Table 7.5 the mean standard deviations for three measurements

Table 7.5 Reproducibility of circumference measurements – mean s.d. of three measurements.

	B-scan	Real-time scan	n	P
Abdomen	0.61 cm	0.70 cm	21	NS
Head	0.33 cm	0.57 cm	20	0.02

did not differ significantly; being 0.61 cm for static scanning and 0.70 cm for real-time scanning. There was no variation in the reproducibility with gestational age. Linear regression confirmed the close correlation between the measurements and the correlation coefficient was 0.998.

The reproducibility of static scan circumference measurements has been studied by Campbell (1976). The mean standard deviation for three measurements in 20 patients was 0.18 cm for the head circumference and 0.30 cm for the abdominal circumference. These figures are approximately half those found in the present study.

Clinical implications

Real-time abdominal circumference measurements appear to be as reproducible as static scan measurements in the hands of average workers, and static scan normal data may be used in interpreting real-time measurements.

The practical use of real-time ultrasound in abdominal circumference measurement is less satisfactory than these figures suggest. The fetal outlines are much less precisely defined than in static scan images and a variable amount of extrapolation is required to obtain a measurement. Greater operator experience is thus required. Static scan equipment offers a wider selection of image ratios which allows the largest possible image to be recorded for measurement. The ADR offers only 1/3, 1/2 and 1/1, the large gap between half the life size means that measurements are usually made at half size —

in contrast to the larger 3/5 or 4/5 static scan images. The measurement of larger images is, of course, more accurate.

Abdominal circumference measurement is playing an increasing role in detecting fetal growth retardation. Campbell and Wilkin (1975), using a computer model, predicted that a single measurement of the fetal abdominal circumference at 32 weeks menstrual age would detect 87% of growth-retarded fetuses. The detection rate fell slightly with advancing gestational age, but was still 75% at 36 weeks. This is significantly better than the results of serial BPD measurement and urinary oestrogen assays reported by Campbell and Kurjak (1972) in which the detection rate was 75% and 53% respectively. Abdominal circumference measurement is also thought to be associated with a lower false-positive rate, i.e. 1% as against 17% for BPD and oestrogen assay.

Clearly these predictions will be less satisfactory when based on less reproducible measurements. Unfortunately Campbell and Wilkin do not provide reproducibility data, and point out that the wider the confidence limits of the measurements, the longer the interval required between measurements before reliable conclusions can be made about a fetus's growth rate. Campbell (1976) calculated that his 95% confidence limits for weekly growth rate assessment were 0.835 cm. The weekly abdominal circumference growth rate is 1.01 cm between 30 and 36 weeks and 0.74 cm between 36 weeks and term. These figures suggest that fortnightly measurements may be clinically meaningful until term. Measurements at longer intervals, as implied by less reproducible measurements, would be of limited use to the clinician. Therefore the problem posed by the present results is how to increase the precision of both techniques in measuring the abdominal circumference.

Static scan precision may be improved by greater attention to the details of the technique, especially in aligning the scanning plane relative to the fetal long axis. (This will neither increase the number of patients who may be examined in a given time nor reduce the need for highly trained operators.) Preliminary experience suggests that more accurate alignment may be obtained by using the fetal abdominal aorta as the reference point, displayed in its full length in a longitudinal scan parallel to the coronal plane. This requires a preliminary transverse scan to determine the coronal plane bearing out the above remarks.

In contrast, technical advances in real-time equipment promise to improve the results obtained in the hands of less experienced operators. The use of a freeze-frame will allow the operator to select the optimum time for measurement, i.e. when the fetus has moved to a position where there is minimal acoustic shadowing and confusion of the fetal outline due to closely applied limbs etc. On-screen measuring systems will enable large images with the maximum grey scaling to be measured immediately, i.e. while the operator's memory of the added clarity of the fetal outlines afforded by movement is still fresh.

Real-time imaging has the advantage that the image is formed over a very short time relative to static scanning. The errors introduced by fetal movement during scanning should therefore be reduced in real-time scanning. However, the inability to compound, that is direct the sound in several directions while the image is being built up, is a serious disadvantage of real-time scanning. This leads to incomplete outlines due to the fetal spine and limbs blocking the sound (acoustic shadowing) and a less precise delineation of the intra-fetal anatomy. This is because the sound cannot be directed at right angles to tissue interfaces in different planes – a prerequisite for producing strong echoes of such important structures as the fetal umbilical vein. Compounding also makes the best use of axial resolution which is superior to the lateral resolution relied on for visualization across the beam in real-time scanning.

MECHANICAL SECTOR SCANNERS

Two prototype mechanical sector scanners have been evaluated briefly in our department. It should be stressed these were prototypes under development by Nuclear Enterprises Ltd. and differ considerably from the production versions. Although we were able to use the equipment for a limited time only, our preliminary results suggest that this equipment is able to achieve a similar level of reproducibility as linear array real-time scanners.

The reproducibility of BPD measurements and head circumference was studied in 12 patients using a Diasonograph 4200 and sector scanner attachment. The results, shown in Table 7.6, demonstrate that the sector scanner reproducibility is within the range reported for linear array scanners.

Table 7.6 Comparative reproducibility of mechanical sector scan and static scan measurement of the BPD and head circumference – mean s.d. of three measurements.

	Sector scan	B-scan	*P*
BPD	1.29 mm	0.62 mm	0.05
HC	0.59 cm	0.45 cm	NS

It is interesting that the reproducibility of the head circumference measurements is not significantly different from that of static scanners. This may be contrasted with the results for linear array real-time scanners, where both the BPD and head circumference were less reproducible. This, together with the excellent delineation of the intra-cerebral anatomy observed with the mechanical sector scanner, lends some support to our clinical impression that the equipment was not achieving its potential accuracy in BPD measurement. This is probably due to the difficulty of conceptualizing the position of the scan plane in space. The design of the transducer gives the operator minimal

proprioceptive clues to the position of the scan plane, particularly when compared to the use of a linear array transducer. Also the scan plane must be
aligned not only relative to the fetal head, but also relative to the caliper
system (Fig. 7.3).

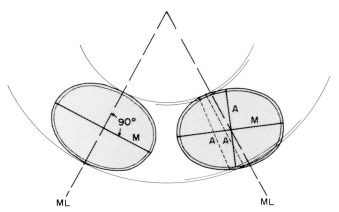

Fig. 7.3   Effect of misorientation of the calipers relative to the fetal head. M   midline
echo – the BPD is measured perpendicular to this; ML   line along which the caliper
is measuring, i.e. a diameter of a circle is centred at the centre of rotation of the transducer; A   various misalignments in attempts to measure the BPD.

In summary, sector scanners seem to be capable of comparable accuracy
to linear array real-time scanners. The provision of a more ergonomic or
functional design of transducer may improve the results obtained with mechanical sector scanners. The ability to apply omnidirectional calipers to a
freeze-frame image would also be helpful.

REFERENCES

CAMPBELL S. (1968) An improved method of fetal cephalometry by ultrasound. *J.
   Obstet. Gynaecol. Br. Cwlth.* **75**, 568.
CAMPBELL S. (1970) Ultrasonic fetal cephalometry during the second trimester of pregnancy. *J. Obstet. Gynaecol. Br. Cwlth.* **77**, 1057.
CAMPBELL S. (1976) Fetal growth. In *Fetal Physiology and Medicine*, eds. R. W. Beard
   and P. W. Nathanielsy, ch. 15. W. B. Saunders, Philadelphia.
CAMPBELL S. & KURJAK A. (1972) Comparison between urinary oestrogen assay and
   serial ultrasonic cephalometry in the assessment of fetal growth retardation *Br.
   med. J.* iv, 337.
CAMPBELL S. & NEWMAN G. B. (1971) Growth of the fetal biparietal diameter during
   normal pregnancy. *J. Obstet. Gynaecol. Br. Cwlth.* **78**, 513.
CAMPBELL S. & WILKIN D. (1975) Ultrasonic measurement of the fetal abdomen circumference in the estimation of fetal weight. *Br. J. Obstet. Gynaecol.* **82**, 689.
COOPERBERG P. L., CHERUB T., KITE V. & AUSTIN S. (1976) Biparietal diameter: A comparison of real time and conventional B scan techniques. *J.C.V.* **4**, 421.

DAVISON J. M., HIRD T., FAIR V. & WHILLINGHAM T. A. (1973) The limitations of ultrasonic fetal cephalometry. *J. Obstet. Gynaecol. Br. Cwlth.* **80,** 769.

DOCKER M. F. & SETTATREE R. S. (1977) Comparison between linear assay real time ultrasonic scanning and conventional compound scanning in the measurement of the fetal biparietal diameter. *Br. J. Obstet. Gynaecol.* **84,** 924.

LUNT, R. M. & CHARD T. (1974) Reproducibility of measurement of the fetal biparietal diameter by ultrasonic cephalometry. *J. Obstet. Gynaecol. Br. Cwlth.* **81,** 682.

ROBINSON H. P. (1973) Sonar measurement of fetal crown–rump length as means of assessing maturity in the first trimester of pregnancy. *Br. med. J.* iv, 28.

VARMA T. R. (1973) Prediction of delivery date by ultrasound cephalometry. *J. Obstet. Gynaecol. Br. Cwlth.* **80,** 316.

WILLOCKS J., DONALD I., DUGGAN T. C. & DAY N. (1964) *J. Obstet. Gynaecol. Br. Cwlth.* **71,** 11.

CHAPTER 8

The dynamics of fetal respiratory movements in man

G. Gennser

Fetal respiratory movements (FRM) have been observed for hundreds of years, in fact since their mention in 'De Humani Corporis Fabrica Libri Septem' by Vesalius in 1543. However, only recently — during the past 6 years — have FRM in man been recorded in such a way that their occurrence *in utero* as a physiological event has been beyond doubt. This achievement followed the observations, made simultaneously by two independent groups, that in chronic fetal lamb preparations irregular intermittent changes in tracheal pressure indicated respiratory activity (Dåwes *et al* 1970, Merlet *et al* 1970). Once the FRM were demonstrated, the chronic preparations of fetal monkey and lamb were found to lend themselves excellently to the study of antenatal respiration. Parameters which directly or indirectly reflect respiration in the fetus are the pressure changes in the fetal trachea and oesophagus, the flow in the fetal trachea, the velocity of the venous return in the great vessels, the movements of the fetal chest and abdominal wall, and the electromyelogram of the fetal diaphragm and intercostal muscles. The great number of studies on FRM in experimental animals have been reviewed by Wilds (1978).

The human fetus, on the other hand, is for obvious reasons far less accessible. It was only with the introduction of a non-invasive ultrasound technique that Boddy and Robinson in 1971 managed to confirm the FRM that Ahlfeld had observed in 1888 using a crude tocographic method. Ultrasonic echofetography has remained the method of choice for detection of FRM in man, using either pulsed ultrasound to follow the movements of the fetal interfaces or the Doppler technique to follow the flow variations in the great veins.

The early studies of human FRM utilized the one-dimensional 'ice-pick' representation provided by the A-mode ultrasound technique. This method has considerable shortcomings, namely in the difficulty of identifying the target (the ultrasonic beam has to be constantly directed through the fetal heart as a means of orientation), in a variety of artefacts (Maršál *et al*), and in requiring a highly skilled operator. Despite several attempts at improving the reliability, the inherent deficiencies of the A-mode technique persisted. When real-time ultrasound B-mode equipment became available, it was rapidly adopted for monitoring of FRM (Gennser & Maršál 1975, Hohler & Fox 1976). This mode is at present widely used for detection of fetal movements, and electronic interfaces have been constructed to supplement the echoscopes for quantitative measurement of movements (Lindström *et al* 1977, Korba *et al*). The usefulness of a continuous-wave Doppler system for monitoring FRM has been evaluated in Oxford. Its detection of fetal breathing is dependent on the identification of the flow velocity changes in the venous return to the fetal chest (Gough & Poore 1977). The time lag between the respiratory and the circulatory events somewhat limits the application of this method for studying the dynamics of the FRM. Reports have recently appeared of studies on FRM in man performed by means of an external tocographic system (Timor-Tritsch *et al* 1976, Timor-Tritsch *et al* 1977). However, this indirect method obviously is less able than ultrasound to detect and distinguish FRM.

The investigations of FRM in man have long been directed to the determination of their presence and to their incidence during different situations and challenges in fetal life. There has been a relative scarcity of quantitative data such as the character of the single breaths and the time course of the breathing events. This lack is in contrast to the early enthusiastic attempts to correlate FRM to clinical states, such as gestational age and fetal well-being. Only recently have serious efforts been made to critically evaluate the use of FRM for clinical purposes (Maršál 1978).

This chapter covers some of the dynamic characteristics of FRM in man, detected and measured by a real-time scanner and a time-distance recorder, and intended to serve as a basis for further comparative studies. As measurements of the amplitude of respiratory movements depend on the fetal section chosen and on the angle of insonation, such a parameter is difficult to evaluate. The chapter therefore concentrates upon the timing of the movements.

METHODS

The equipment at the Laboratory for Fetal Breathing at the Maternity Unit has been developed during several years in collaboration with the Department of Biomedical Engineering. The principles have been to produce means for quantitatively measuring the fetal movements with a high degree of reliability and resolution. At present, this is achieved by the following components (Fig. 8.1):

1 A *real-time ultrasound scanner* for detection of the FRM is the central part of the equipment. From the outset a scanner which utilizes a rotating transducer and mirror optics for sectional insonation of the object by a parallel moving ultrasound beam (Vidoson 635, Siemens) was used. This equipment yields a two-dimensional B-mode image of 140 lines with a cross-

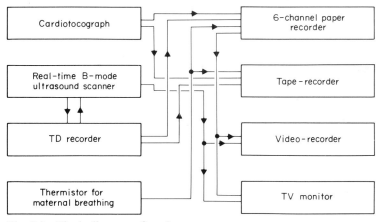

Fig. 8.1   Block diagram of equipment.

section 14 cm × 16 cm displayed 16 times/sec. Since 1977 this has been used alternately with a real-time scanner with grey-scale facilities and fitted with a linear array transducer containing 64 elements operated at a frequency of 3.5 MHz (Advances Diagnostic Research Corporation). The image of a cross-sectional area 17 cm × 20 cm is formed by 60 image lines with a frequency of 40 frames/sec.

2   For measuring the fetal trunk movements, visually identified as respiratory movements, a *time–distance* (*TD*) *recorder* (Krantzbühler & Sohn) is used as an interface (Lindström *et al* 1977). This device works by measuring the movements, relative to each other, of two echoes displayed on the echoscope screen. Any of the real-time image lines can be chosen for measurement, and the two echoes are selected by markers. The instantaneous distance between the two echoes provides an analog output signal and is indicated on the echoscope screen as a brightness-intensified part of the image line.

As the echo-signals from deeper fetal structures are occasionally not strong enough to be gated by the instrument, artefactual spikes might occur in the output voltage. To eliminate this noise, the TD recorder is fitted with a non-linear, analog, slow-rate filter with a voltage rate corresponding to movements of 30 mm/sec. This type of filter has the advantage of minimal distortion of phase and amplitude, when the slow-rate limit is not exceeded. A signal-clearing indicator unit informs the operator when the filter is activated. The signal from this unit, which most often coincides with gross fetal movements, is valuable for indicating when the output voltage is contaminated by filtered transients.

3   It has been recognized that maternal breathing movements are prone to influence the ultrasonic recording and are an important source of artefactual signals (Maršál *et al*). Maternal breathing is therefore regularly recorded via a *nasal thermistor* in order to facilitate the identification of maternal movements transmitted to the fetal trunk.

4   The fetal heart rate is frequently monitored by using a conventional external fetal *electrocardiograph* (Hewlett–Packard).

5   The output signals from the measuring devices are recorded on a 6-channel *polygraph* (Watanabe) using a paper speed of 100 mm/min. Most examinations are performed for at least 30 minutes.

6   The image displayed on the scanner screen is transferred to a 19 inch *video monitor* and representative sequences are recorded on a *video recorder* (VCR N1520, Philips) supplied with a freeze-frame replay unit. A split-image device allows the section of the tracings being recorded on the polygraph to be simultaneously displayed in the ultrasonic image on the monitor screen and to be stored on the video tape. This arrangement facilitates the supervision of the recording and guarantees a correct time correlation of the measured signals with the events detected by the echoscope.

The experience gained at the Laboratory for Fetal Breathing can be seen in the type of demands for equipment and the technical solutions therefore produced over several years (Table 8.1).

Table 8.1   Investigator's demands and their satisfaction.

Requirement	Reason	Technical solution
Full visualization of the fetal trunk	Identification of FRM; selecting optimal part for insonation of the fetal trunk.	Ultrasonic real-time B-mode scanner
Perpetual supervision of the fetus	Excluding artefacts. Recognition of factors influencing FRM	Ultrasonic real-time B-mode scanner
Automatic measurements of FRM	Quantification of FRM	TD recorder
Measuring changes of a diameter of fetal trunk cross-section	Minimizing influence of non-specific movements	Differential measurement by TD recorder

More than 350 examinations — mostly on hospital patients — have been performed with the present equipment. The data presented here are from women without any clinical signs of a compromised fetus. The recordings were made for at least 30 minutes with the women supine. Only when a patient expressed discomfort or when signs of the hypotension syndrome became evident, was she tilted 20°–30° to her left.

After an initial survey for orientation of the fetal position, the examiner chooses a longitudinal section as close as possible to the median plane. The breathing excursions are usually of greatest amplitude in the abdominal wall, and the recordings have therefore been made as a rule with the TD recorder gating a point of the anterior body outline at the umbilical level. The site of measurement is also significant for the identification of the respiratory phase. As the majority of FRM are of a paradoxical nature (see below), the outward movement of the abdominal wall signals an inspiratory-like part of the respiratory cycle. This phase is characterized by a retraction of the chest wall, which is therefore 180° out of phase with the abdominal wall (see below).

SYNCHRONY OF FRM

Real-time B-mode scanners have made it possible to study in detail the echo images of fetal respiratory activity. The sequence of movements during a cycle of breathing has been thoroughly described by Maršál (1978) and Bots (1977). The central event is evidently the contraction of the diaphragm, which increases the intra-abdominal pressure and pushes the abdominal wall outwards, at the same time retracting the chest wall. The movements of the abdominal and chest walls are therefore out of phase or paradoxical. This is the pattern generally observed on the scanner screen (Maršál 1978, Patrick *et al* 1978). However, a more detailed analysis of the relative time sequence of the movements was achieved by replay and measurement of the events stored on videotape, and by comparing the simultaneous signals of chest wall and abdominal wall movements obtained by *two* TD recorders attached to the same scanner (Gennser 1978). Such a study revealed that the pattern of paradoxical breathing is not a constant one, even in the same train of continuous breathing. Although the majority of all breathing movements observed are of this see-saw type, a few breaths occur with the trunk wall movements *in phase* with each other (Fig. 8.2). Furthermore, the position of the 'hinge' between the chest wall and the abdominal wall seems at times to be at different levels (Gennser 1978). A variable movement pattern in fetal lambs was also recently shown using sets of ultrasound transducers attached to the fetal body (Poore, *pers. commun.*). The contraction of the intercostal muscles, which is the main stabilizing factor of the rib cage in young individuals, is largely inhibited during antenatal life, as judged by an inactive intercostal EMG in fetal lambs (Hardin *et al* 1977). These findings have several implications for the interpretation of the FRM image produced by pulsed ultrasound.

1   The pattern of see-saw breathing suggests that the fetal respiration in man is predominantly isovolumic, i.e. the total volume of the fetus is not altered by the respiratory movements. This concept implies that pressure changes in the fetal chest, caused by the contraction of the diaphragm, are largely

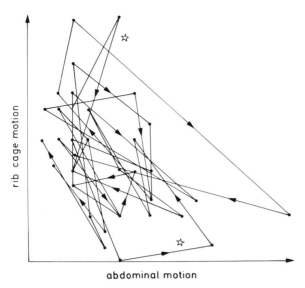

Fig. 8.2   X–Y display of relative lengths of antero-posterior diameter of rib cage and abdomen during successive fetal breaths. The majority of the breathing movements are paradoxical; in two breaths (indicated) the motion components are in phase. Gestational age 38 weeks.

taken up by the retraction of the unstable chest walls and, consequently, little or no flow occurs in the fetal respiratory tract. The observation by Dawes and co-workers (1972) that the respiratory movements in fetal lambs are associated with only small movements of tracheal fluid indirectly supports this idea.

2 The variability of the movement pattern observed by ultrasound reflects the instability of the pliable fetal chest wall. It suggests that any change of the fetal rib cage shape in one sectional plane (i.e. during the occasional unidirectional movements of the fetal chest and abdomen) might, with regard to its effect on the chest volume, be counteracted by reverse movements in another plane. There is thus at present no firm ultrasonic evidence that any human FRM is in fact changing the chest volume and thereby causing an increased tracheal flow. It seems that the activity of the intercostal muscles and their effect on the rib cage stability might play a critical role in whether the breathing movements will induce a flow in the fetal respiratory tract. Present observations provide indirect evidence that intercostal muscle activity is generally inhibited during FRM in man. This hypothesis is supported by the fact that breathing movements in fetal lambs coincide with REM-sleep (Dawes *et al* 1972) and that, in infants, distortion of rib cage motion occurs during REM-sleep (Knill *et al* 1976).

TIME CHARACTERISTICS OF SINGLE BREATHS

The breathing movements in the human fetus are episodic and irregular in time, in this respect resembling the fetal breathing in sheep (Dawes *et al* 1972). The human FRM appears as sequences of breaths lasting 57.7 ± 6.2 sec. (mean $\pm$ SEM), interspersed by periods of apnea and gross fetal movements lasting 66.3 ± 8.1 sec. These data, obtained from 5 pregnant women being monitored four times daily for 5 consecutive days, accord well with the observations by Patrick *et al* (1978) made on 10 women monitored for eight hours continuously. The average frequency of breathing movements varies widely even during periods of continuous breathing (range 35–70 breaths/ min.) (Maršál 1978) with occasional fast rates up to 200 breaths/min (Patrick *et al* 1978). Because of these variations, the average rate of respiration is dependent on the length of the time base and is therefore probably less meaningful than the instantaneous breath-to-breath interval (see below).

During the trains of successive breaths, the duration of the active phase occupies most of the respiration cycle (Table 8.2). In five apparently healthy fetuses of 36–38 weeks gestational age, this amounted to $88.9 \pm 4.4\%$. This relative duration of the active breathing phase exceeds that previously reported (Bots 1977) and can probably be ascribed to the high range resolution of the present measuring technique. The ratio between inspiratory time and expiratory time varies somewhat inter- and intra-fetally (see Table 8.2), but for each epoch of continuous respiration a linear relation exists between the inspiratory period and the total active breathing phase (Fig. 8.3). A similar correlation has been demonstrated in neonates (Olinsky 1974) and suggests that the duration of expiration is determined by the preceding inspiratory time.

The duration of the breath-to-breath intervals shows, on average, a rather small scatter (see Table 8.2). A finer analysis of the intervals was performed by means of an electronic device based upon a phase-locked loop principle (Stagg & Gennser 1978). This renders it possible to detect, within a given frequency range, a signal that is submerged even in high-amplitude noise.

Table 8.2 Parameters of a single episode of continuous fetal respiration in 5 fetuses (gestational age 36–38 weeks). Mean $\pm$ SEM.

Fetus	Number of cycles	Duration of active breathing movement, sec.	Inspiration time/ expiration time, ratio	Breath-to-breath interval, sec.
EO	56	1.28 ± 0.03	1.20 ± 0.04	1.33 ± 0.03
BO	46	1.00 ± 0.02	0.79 ± 0.05	1.05 ± 0.01
BP	50	1.22 ± 0.03	1.26 ± 0.05	1.29 ± 0.02
ER	20	0.97 ± 0.02	0.81 ± 0.08	1.33 ± 0.04
BS	42	0.87 ± 0.03	1.26 ± 0.11	1.02 ± 0.04

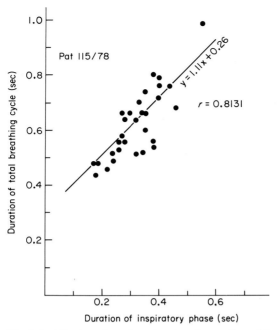

Fig. 8.3 The duration of total active phase of breathing cycle in relation to the duration of inspiration. Values from one train of successive breaths. Gestational age 37 weeks.

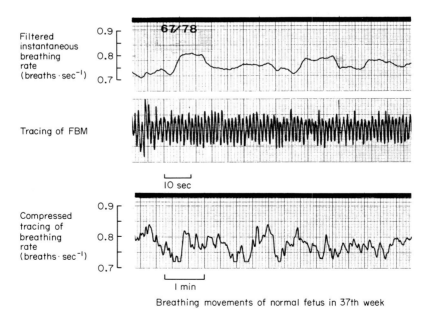

Breathing movements of normal fetus in 37th week

Fig. 8.4 Fetal breathing movements registered from normal fetus in the 37th week via a TD recorder (middle trace) with the simultaneous, filtered instantaneous breathing rate (top trace). Lower trace depicts the instantaneous breathing rate of the same fetus for a longer period containing a slow undulation frequency of 0.78 cycles per minute.

Processing the output signals from the TD recorder with this device demonstrated fluctuations of the intantaneous breathing rate with obvious periodicity (Fig. 8.4). The cyclic variability of this breathing parameter suggests a regulating system operating *in utero*.

Already the direct viewing of the echo images on the real-time scanner screen has revealed a superficial similarity between continuous FRM and the breathing movements of infants born pre-term. Several of the reported fetal single-breath characteristics show a resemblance to the corresponding

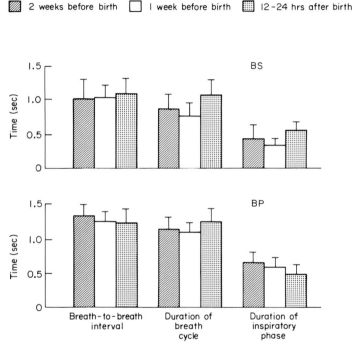

Fig. 8.5 Comparison of breath characteristics in two fetuses (BS and BP, delivered in 37th and 40th week, respectively) at two weeks before birth, one week before birth, and 12–24 hours after birth, respectively. Means and SEM.

parameters of the breathing movements in the neonatal period. Examples of this similarity are given in Fig. 8.5, which compares breathing data of two infants before and after birth. The similarity is remarkable in view of the obvious differences between the pre- and the postnatal systems, e.g. the contents of the airways, the compliance of the lungs and the operational state of the feed-back regulating system involving the chemoreceptors. It is conceivable that further comparisons of fetal and neonatal breathing, taking into consideration the known differences in external circumstances between the two, might shed some light on the intra-uterine regulation of breathing.

RELATION TO FETAL HEART RATE AND ACTIVITY STATE

Both in sheep fetuses (Dalton *et al* 1977) and monkey fetuses (Martin *et al* 1974) a relationship between FRM and heart rate has been demonstrated. Recently, the appearance of a respiratory sinus arrhythmia in the human fetus was reported (Timor-Tritsch *et al* 1977). Wheeler has added to this, the observation in pregnant women of an increased variability of the fetal heart rate during periods of fetal respiration compared with times of apnea. FRM were accompanied by an increase in the standard deviation of the heart beat intervals and an increase in the mean absolute beat-by-beat difference (Wheeler *et al* 1978). These effects have been interpreted as being due to the influence of the respiratory and vasomotor centres of the central nervous system (Timor-Tritsch *et al* 1977). However, experience gained from animal fetuses suggests that peripheral control mechanisms might also be involved (Wheeler *et al* 1978).

Ultrasound shows that the respiratory movements and the gross body movements of the human fetus occur episodically. The two kinds of episodes are, however, not correlated in time, nor in their duration (unpublished observation). Patrick has reported that the incidence of gross movements is independent of that of FRM and postulated that the two functions have different control mechanisms (Patrick *et al* 1978). Wheeler, defining periods of fetal rest exceeding 5 minutes by a decrease in the average fetal heart rate, a decrease in heart rate variation and an absence of gross fetal movements, could not find any association between FRM and the fetal rest–activity cycles (Wheeler *et al* 1978). It might be, however, that some character of FRM, e.g. the variability in the rate of fetal breathing, is determined by the state of fetal activity (Stagg & Gennser 1978).

CONCLUSION

1   The movements of the fetal rib cage and abdominal wall as part of human fetal respiratory movements can be measured with high resolution and freedom from artefacts by a combination of an ultrasound real-time B-mode scanner and a TD recorder. The analog output signal is suitable for timing the breathing events.
2   The human FRM are predominantly paradoxical but show some variation of pattern. The instability of the fetal chest walls suggests inhibited intercostal muscles and makes it virtually impossible to come to any firm conclusions regarding tracheal flow.
3   The active breathing phase occupies most of the respiratory cycle time.
4   The instantaneous breathing rate shows a cyclic variability.
5   Several respiratory cycle parameters in the fetus closely resemble those in the neonatal period.

6 The FRM markedly influences the fetal heart rate variability, presumably both by central and peripheral mechanisms. No association has been found at present between the FRM and the fetal state of rest–activity.

7 It can be expected that the time characteristics of the fetal respiration will be utilized for further evaluation of what causes the fetus to make breathing movements *in utero*, and for renewed attempts to correlate the FRM to the current state of fetal health.

Acknowledgements

This project has, in various parts, been supported by grants from the Swedish Medical Research Council (B79–17X–04517–05A), the Magnus Bergvall Foundation, and the Medical Faculty of the University of Lund. Skilful technical assistance was given by Miss Ann-Charlotte Thuring and Mr Arne Bjuvholt.

REFERENCES

AHLFELD F. (1888) Ueber bisher noch nicht beschriebene intrauterine Bewegungen des Kindes. *Verh. dtsch. Ges. Gynäk.*, Zweiter Kongress, 203. Breitkopf und Härtel, Leipzig.

BODDY K. & ROBINSON J. (1971) External method for detection of fetal breathing movements in utero. *Lancet* ii, 1231.

BOTS R. S. G. M. (1977) Investigation of breathing movements of the human foetus, application of the multiscan/M-mode echography (Dutch, with English summary). Thesis, Vrije Universiteit te Amsterdam.

DALTON K. J., DAWES G. S. & PATRICK J. (1977) Diurnal, respiratory and other rhythms of fetal heart rate in lambs. *Am. J. Obstet. Gynecol.* **127**, 414.

DAWES G. S., FOX H. E., LEDUC B. M., LIGGINS G. C. & RICHARDS R. T. (1970) Respiratory movements and paradoxical sleep in the foetal lamb. *J. Physiol.* **210**, 47P.

DAWES G. S., FOX H. E., LEDUC B. M., LIGGINS G. C. & RICHARDS R. T. (1972) Respiratory movements and rapid eye movement sleep in the foetal lambs. *J. Physiol.* **220**, 119.

GENNSER G. (1978) The synchrony of fetal breathing movements in man.

GENNSER G. & MARŠÁL K. (1975) Fetal breathing movements in man. Film presented at the 2nd Conference on Fetal Breathing, Nuffield Institute for Medical Research, Oxford.

GOUGH J. D. & POORE R. (1977) Directional Doppler measurements of foetal breathing. *J. Physiol.* **272**, 12P.

HARDIN R., JOHNSON P., McCLELLAND M. E., McLEOD C. N. & WHYTE P. L. (1977) Laryngeal function during breathing and swallowing in foetal and newborn lambs. *J. Physiol.* **272**, 14P.

HOHLER C. W. & FOX H. E. (1976) Real-time gray-scale B-scan ultrasound recording of human fetal breathing movements *in utero*. In *Ultrasound in Medicine*, eds D. N. White and R. Barnes, p. 203. Plenum, New York.

KNILL R., ANDREWS W., BRYAN A. C. & BRYAN M. H. (1976) Respiratory load compensation in infants. *J. Appl. Physiol.* **40**, 357.

KORBA L. W., COUSIN A. J., COBBOLD R. S. C. & GARE, D. An ultrasonic fetal respiratory movement monitor. In Press.

LINDSTRÖM K., MARŠÁL K., GENNSER, G., BENGTSSON L., BENTHIN M. & DAHL P. (1977) Device for measurement of fetal breathing movements—I The TD-recorder. A new system for recording the distance between two echogenerating structures as a function of time. *Ultrasound Med. Biol.* **3**, 143.

MARŠÁL K. (1978) Fetal breathing movements in man — characteristics and clinical significance. *Obstet. Gynecol.*

MARŠÁL K., GENNSER G., LINDSTRÖM K. & ULMSTEN U. Errors and pitfalls in ultrasonic measurements of fetal breathing movements. In *International Symposium on Ultrasound Diagnosis*, eds A. Kurjak, B. Breyer and V. Latin. Elsevier, Amsterdam. In Press.

MARTIN C. B. Jr., MURATA Y., PETRIE R. H. & PARER J. T. (1974) Respiratory movements in fetal rhesus monkeys. *Am. J. Obstet. Gynecol.* **119**, 939.

MERLET C., HOERTER J., DEVILLENEUVE CH. & TCHOBROUTSKY C. (1970) Mise en évidence de movements respiratoires chez le foetus d'agneau *in utero* au cours du dernier mois de la gestation. *C.R. Acad. Sc. Paris* **270**, 2462.

OLINSKY A., BRYAN M. H. & BRYAN A. C. (1974) Influence of lung inflation on respiratory control in neonates. *J. Appl. Physiol.* **36**, 426.

PATRICK J., FETHERSTON W., VICK H. & VOEGELIN R. (1978) Human fetal breathing movements and gross fetal body movements at weeks 34 to 35 of gestation. *Am. J. Obstet. Gynecol.* **130**, 693.

STAGG J. & GENNSER G. (1978) Electronic analysis of foetal breathing movements. A practical analysis of phase-lock-loop principles. *Biomed. Engineering.*

TIMOR-TRITSCH I., ZADOR I., HERTZ R. H. & ROSEN M. G. (1976) Classification of human fetal movement. *Am. J. Obstet. Gynecol.* **126**, 70.

TIMOR-TRITSCH I., ZADOR I., HERTZ R. H. & ROSEN M. G. (1977) Human fetal respiratory arrhythmia. *Am. J. Obstet. Gynecol.* **127**, 662.

WHEELER T., GENNSER G., MURRILLS A. J. & LINDVALL A. (1978) Combined recordings of fetal breathing and fetal heart rate in the human. Transactions of 5th Conference on Fetal Breating, Nijmegen.

WILDS P. L. (1978) Observations of intrauterine fetal breathing movements — A review. *Am. J. Obstet. Gynecol.* **131**, 315.

CHAPTER 9

The effect of drugs on fetal breathing movements

P. J. Lewis & Elena Olivier

The study of the effect of drugs on human fetal breathing movements is of interest for a variety of reasons.

1 *Scientific interest.* The intact human fetus *in utero* is relatively inaccessible and very few measurements of the effect of drugs can be carried out in this situation. Indeed it is only heart rate, whole body movements and placental hormone production which can be measured and observation of fetal breathing adds another variable to this short list. Observing the effect of drugs on these fetal variables might be a means of studying transfer of drugs into the fetus and the speed at which this occurs in different pathological conditions.

2 *Development of drug therapy.* It is entirely possible that in the future clinicians might wish to stop or start fetal breathing activity in the fetus as a therapeutic goal. For example, it is known that diabetic fetuses make more and earlier breathing movements than do normal fetuses and it is a possibility that this alteration in breathing activity changes the distribution of pulmonary surfactant between amniotic fluid and the lung. If fetal breathing activity was reduced to normal in these fetuses, interpretation of amniotic lecithin to sphingomyelin ratios might be easier. More importantly, stimulation of fetal breathing in fetuses at risk of poor pulmonary development such as those with oligo-hydramnios might aid lung development. If precise control of fetal breathing were available pharmacologically, then aspiration of meconium by the fetus might be prevented.

3 *Tests of fetal function.* Several workers have suggested that fetal breathing movements might be useful as a test of fetal function. Because of this it is obviously important that the influence of any medication the mother might be given, such as anti-hypertensives or sedatives, should be known and allowance made when the results of these tests are considered.

4 *Tests of analgesics.* It has been suggested that human fetal breathing activity is closely related to central nervous activity in the fetus although in man there is no way this relationship can be confirmed at present. However, if this is indeed the case, then observation of the effect of different analgesics and sedative agents on fetal breathing could provide us with a sensitive in-vivo test system for ranking the different analgesic drugs which are used in labour. In this way a rational basis for deciding what is a good and bad analgesic for use at delivery would be at last be available.

Despite these good reasons for investigating the effect of drugs on fetal breathing, it must be admitted at the outset that the study is still in its early stages and none of the above goals can yet be satisfied. Indeed, it seems that fetal breathing research is about to go through a period of disillusionment; it is unlikely that fetal breathing will be established as a useful test of fetal function as the range of normal variability is so great. Part of the problem with fetal breathing has been the inadequacy of the methods for measuring it. With the advent of real-time scanning a lot of these difficulties have disappeared, but there is still not enough emphasis on quantitative measurements.

PHYSIOLOGY OF FETAL BREATHING

Some extrapolations from what is known of the physiology of fetal breathing can help pharmacological investigations. Many factors, some interrelated, have been found to be associated with changes in the frequency or duration of fetal breathing movements in animals and humans. Some of these factors are listed in Table 9.1.

In general fetal breathing seems to be a reflection of central nervous system activity in the fetus. The original work by Dawes and his colleagues at Oxford demonstrated that, in the sheep, coordinated fetal breathing occurs mainly during central nervous system arousal in the fetus, the stage of rapid eye movement sleep (Dawes 1974). The fetus does not breathe continuously but intermittently. There is, however, some confusion about this association of fetal breathing and fetal arousal since, although the amount of coordinated breathing increases progressively during gestation, the proportion of time that the fetus spends in REM sleep probably decreases. There is no evidence that fetal breathing is associated with a particular sleep state in humans.

Table 9.1   Factors known or believed to influence the incidence of human fetal breathing movements.

Gestational age of fetus
Well-being of fetus
Time of day
Maternal blood glucose
Maternal diabetes mellitus
Maternal $PaCO_2$ and PaO_2
Maternal exercise
Maternal drug therapy

However, it is probable from these considerations that any drug which sedates or arouses the fetal central nervous system will change the frequency of fetal breathing.

Another physiological variable which influences fetal breathing is the level of maternal and fetal blood glucose. Hypoglycaemia inhibits fetal breathing in lamb fetuses and oral glucose stimulates fetal breathing in human pregnancy (Lewis *et al* 1978). Hence another pharmacological way of altering fetal breathing would be to alter carbohydrate metabolism in the fetus.

Animal pharmacology

All quantitative work on the animal pharmacology of fetal breathing has been carried out in sheep, usually in chronic preparations in which the fetal trachea was catheterized. Boddy *et al* (1978) carried out a careful study of the effect of small doses of pentobarbitone (4 mg/kg i.v.) given to sheep in the third trimester. This small dose of barbiturate had little apparent effect on the ewe, but markedly diminished fetal breathing movements. The effect of a single dose lasted approximately 2 hours and coincided with a change to high voltage pattern in the fetal electrocorticogram. The time to arrest of fetal breathing — following administration of the pentobarbitone — varied with gestational age. It is interesting that, in similar experiments, doses of pethidine (1–3 mg/kg) had no consistent effect on fetal breathing movements. However, when fetal breathing had been augmented by inducing maternal hypercapnoea, subsequent dosing with pethidine reduced breathing by the fetus.

Condorelli and Scarpelli (1976) in similar experiments also reported that various barbiturates injected into the fetus and into the ewe stopped respiratory movements by sheep fetuses in late gestation.

Piercy *et al* (1977) studied the effects of diazepam. Maternal intravenous infusion of diazepam in a dose of 0.18–0.22 mg/kg reduced the incidence of fetal breathing movements. The time course of this reduction was reproducible and breathing returned to pre-injection levels about 60 minutes after dosing. These authors also studied the effects of caffeine and doxapram. Both these drugs stimulated fetal breathing. When caffeine 1.5–5 mg/kg was administered directly to the fetus, fetal breathing was transiently stimulated for 3–5 minutes. Doxapram also initiated fetal breathing when given directly to the fetus in a dose of 1–2 mg/kg.

Hogg *et al* (1977) also reported that maternal infusion of doxapram stimulated fetal breathing movements in the sheep.

Human pharmacology

Maršál *et al* (1975) investigated 29 pregnant women between the 29th and 35th week of pregnancy who were at risk of pre-term delivery. Nineteen of these women were treated with 12 mg betamethazone daily while 10 served as controls. The incidence of fetal breathing movements was similar in both control and treated groups, implying that the steroid had no effect on fetal breathing activity and that its effect, if any, on surfactant production is mediated by other mechanisms.

Manning *et al* (1975) studied 19 women with uncomplicated pregnancies between the 32nd and 38th week. They showed that smoking two cigarettes caused a marked fall in the proportion of time that the fetal breathing movements were observed. The effect lasted for up to two hours.

In further experiments Manning and Feyerabend (1976) showed that the fall in fetal breathing movements was significantly related to the rise in maternal plasma nicotine after smoking, but not to the rise in carboxyhaemoglobin. The effect of the nicotine was thought to be placental rather than fetal since nicotine given to fetal lambs stimulated breathing rather than depressed it.

Gennser *et al* (1976) reported results of administering a variety of drugs to pregnant women. Pethidine, 1 mg/kg, given to a group of 5 women before the onset of labour caused a decrease of about 50% in fetal breathing movements. In addition the group reported several individual records of the effect of intravenous and intramuscular injections of diazepam. These had little effect on the incidence of fetal breathing. One case of terbutaline infusion to a woman in labour is also reported. This decreased the incidence of apnoeic periods, i.e. stimulated fetal breathing. Finally, these authors presented results to show that cigarette smoking and chewing nicotine-containing gum decreased fetal breathing activity.

Boddy (1977) reviewed the effect of maternal drug administration in human fetal breathing and presented some original data on the effect of barbiturate, diazepam and promazine on women with pre-eclampsia. Intramuscular diazepam (10–20 mg) caused a marked fall in fetal breathing movements, while oral amylobarbitone had little effect. Boddy also reported that methyl dopa diminished fetal breathing movements in some women to whom it was given but this was not a consistent effect.

With the exception of Gennser's study on betamethazone, these human studies have not included control or placebo experiments and, since fetal breathing is not a stable activity, it is possible that some of these drug effects might have been due to the lapse of time or to the psychological effects of the mother being alarmed or reassured by the treatment she was receiving. Most of these preliminary studies have been carried out on patients actually being treated with the substance under investigation and were in the nature of incidental observations. However, most of the results in human pregnancy accord well with the concept developed in sheep, namely that central nervous system depressants decrease fetal breathing while respiratory stimulants increase it.

EXPERIMENTAL STUDIES

The authors have investigated several substances in normal human pregnancy for their effect on fetal breathing and these results are, as yet, unpublished elsewhere. Parameters such as time of day, gestation, maternal
blood glucose level and placebo effects have all been controlled. The only
disadvantage of working in a controlled way with normal patients is that
practical and ethical considerations limit the amount of sedative drugs which
can be given to an ambulant woman in late pregnancy.

In all cases a quantitative method of recording fetal breathing activity
was employed (Campbell *et al* 1977). The fetal chest was visualized in a
sagittal longitudinal section using an ADR 2130 real-time scanner. The image
was videotaped and analysed by a trained observer who depressed a key on
a purpose-built tachometer whenever the fetus made a breath or began or
ended a trunk movement. The tachometer is a modified computer tape punch
in which an internal time clock has been incorporated, its output recording
each event and elapsed time at which the event occurred.

The reproducibility of the observer in estimating the duration of continuous fetal breathing was checked in preliminary experiments. The coefficient of variation was 6.2%.

The first study concerns the effect of small doses of pethidine and diazepam on fetal breathing movements. The protocol for this study was to take
normal, non-smoking women in their first pregnancy between the 34th and
36th week of gestation. These women attended the laboratory on two
occasions within a week. They attended fasting and were given 25 g of glucose
to drink. Fifteen minutes after this dose a half-hour recording of fetal
breathing activity was made and subsequently analysed. After the half-hour
control period, women received in a double-blind manner either intravenous
drug or intravenous saline. A further half-hour period of observation was
then made. Six women in the study received saline and diazepam and six
received saline and pethidine. The proportion of time that the fetus spent
making continuous breathing movements (i.e. intervals between breaths less
than 6 seconds) was calculated, as was the proportion of time the fetus spent
making whole body movements.

Diazepam had no discernible effect on either fetal breathing or fetal movements in the dose used, a bolus injection of 2 mg (Fig. 9.1).

The results of the pethidine study (Fig. 9.2) show that 5 mg intravenous
pethidine has no discernible effect on either fetal activity. These two studies
also indicate that there is little placebo effect; intravenous saline has no consistent effect on either fetal activity.

Ethanol is another central nervous depressant whose effect we have investigated. Fox and co-workers (1978) reported that drinking of 30 ml vodka
by pregnant women suppressed fetal breathing almost to zero within 30
minutes of ingestion. Lewis and Boylan (unpublished findings) have studied
the effect of 40 ml vodka, containing 15 ml of ethanol, on fetal breathing in

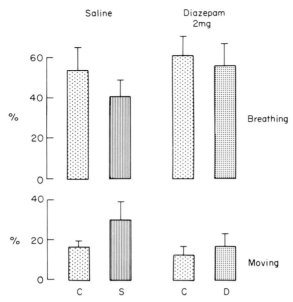

Fig. 9.1   Effect of intravenous diazepam (2 mg) or saline on the (mean ± SEM) proportion of time fetuses spend breathing and moving.

6 normal pregnant women between the 34th and 36th week of gestation. A double-blind design was used and each woman had fetal breathing measurements made on two occasions, once after receiving vodka and the other after receiving orange juice alone. The mean fetal breathing index was reduced

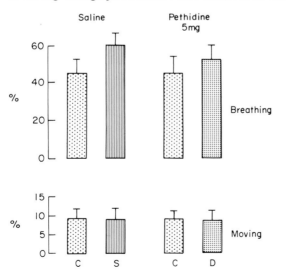

Fig. 9.2   Effect of intravenous pethidine (5 mg) or saline on the (mean ± SEM) proportion of time fetuses spend breathing and moving.

from 51% to 46% after orange, but from 41% to 14% after ethanol, a significant reduction due to the active drug.

We looked next at some respiratory stimulants using somewhat different design. Since the previous work had shown that placebo injections had no effect on fetal breathing activity, placebo was not included. Normal primiparous non-smoking women between 34 and 38 weeks were also investigated. They were, however, investigated fasting and no glucose was given to them during the course of the experiment. Base-line fetal breathing measurements were made for 30 minutes. They were then given salbutamol either 4 mg or 8 mg orally and half-hour recordings were made from 30 to 60 minutes after dosing and from 90 to 120 minutes after dosing. Six patients were studied for each dose. Salbutamol was investigated for three reasons; first because the work of Gennser suggests that terbutaline, another β-mimetic compound, had a stimulatory effect on fetal breathing; secondly because stimulation of β-1 receptors increases respiratory rate in adults, and thirdly because salbutamol is a mildly hyperglycaemic agent.

Fig. 9.3 shows that salbutamol, either 4 mg or 8 mg, had no effect on either fetal breathing activity or fetal movements. This is quite surprising since it is often stated by obstetricians that, when women are given 8 mg doses of

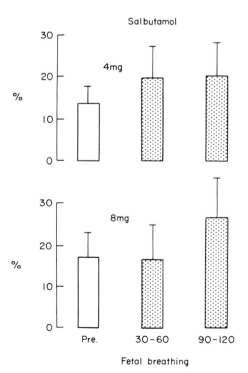

Fig. 9.3   Effect of either 4 mg or 8 mg oral salbutamol on the (mean ± SEM) proportion of time fetuses spend breathing.

salbutamol, they often complain of excessive fetal movement. This may be another illustration of the difference between the activity of normal and compromised fetuses.

Finally, we have investigated the effect on 6 patients of 50 mg of caffeine given orally in a similar designed study; this too had no effect on fetal movements.

CONCLUSION

Our conclusions from these studies on human fetal breathing and the effect of drugs are firstly that the human fetus is not as sensitive to CNS depressant drugs as has been often thought. Secondly, we would question some of the data obtained from less well controlled studies on depressants in human pregnancy. In the normal fetus it seems that fetal breathing is a stable activity much more influenced by maternal plasma glucose than by sedative or stimulant drugs.

Acknowledgements

These studies were supported by grants from the Wellcome Trust, the Cilag-Chemie Foundation for Therapeutic Research and Action Research for the Crippled Child. Some were carried out in collaboration with Stuart Campbell and Alistair Roberts. E. Olivier was sponsored by a studentship of the Fundacion Gran Marischal de Aijacucho, Venezuela.

REFERENCES

BODDY K. (1977) The Influence of Maternal Drug Administration on Human Fetal Breathing Movements *in utero*. In *Therapeutic Problems in Pregnancy*, ed. P. J. Lewis, p. 153. MTP, Lancaster.

BODDY K., DAWES G. S., FISCHER R. L., PINTER S. & ROBINSON J. S. (1978) The effects of pentobarbitone and pethidine on foetal breathing movements in sheep. *Br. J. Pharmacol.* **57**, 311.

CAMPBELL S., FRIEDMAN L. A., LEWIS P. J., TALBERT D. G. & THOMS A. (1977) Recording foetal breathing in man. *Br. J. Pharmacol.* **59**, 533P.

CONDORELLI S. & SCARPELLI E. M. (1976) Fetal breathing: Induction *in utero* and effects of vagotomy and barbiturate. *J. Pediatr.* **88**, 94.

DAWES G. S. (1974) Breathing before birth in animals and man. *N. Eng. J. Med.* **290**, 557.

FOX H. E., STEINBRECHER M., PESSEL D., INGLIS J., MEDVID L. & ANGEL, E. (1978) Maternal ethanol ingestion and the occurrence of human fetal breathing movements. *Am. J. Obstet. Gynecol.* **132**, 354.

GENNSER G., MARŠÁL K. & LINDSTRÖM K. (1976) Influence of External Factors on Breathing Movements in the Human Fetus. Proceedings 5th European Congress on Perinatal Medicine, p. 181.

HOGG M. I. J., GOLDING R. H. & ROSEN M. (1977) The effect of doxapram on fetal breathing in the sheep. *Br. J. Obstet. Gynaecol.* **84**, 48.

LEWIS P. J., TRUDINGER B. J. & MANGEZ J. (1978) Effect of maternal glucose ingestion on fetal breathing and body movements in late pregnancy. *Br. J. Obstet. Gynaecol.* **85**, 86.

MANNING F. A. & FEYERABEND C. (1976) Cigarette smoking and fetal breathing movements. *Br. J. Obstet. Gynaecol.* **83**, 262.

MANNING F., WYN-PUGH E. & BODDY K. (1975) Effect of cigarette smoking on fetal breathing movements in normal pregnancies. *Br. med. J.* i, 552.

MARŠÁL K. S., GENNSER G. M. & OHRLANDER S. A. V. (1975) Fetal and neonatal breathing movements in man after betamethazone. *Life Sciences* **17**, 449.

PIERCY W. N., DAY M. A., NEIMS A. H. & WILLIAMS R. L. (1977) Alteration of ovine fetal respiratory-like activity by diazepam, caffeine and doxapram. *Am. J. Obstet. Gynecol.* **127**, 43.

CHAPTER 10

Fetal activity in normal and growth-retarded fetuses

A. B. Roberts, D. J. Little, D. Cooper & S. Campbell

The recent development of good resolution real-time ultrasound scanners means that fetal activity can at last be studied in detail. In the past, assumptions about fetal movement have been made by more indirect methods. These included maternal perception of fetal movement (Pearson & Weaver 1976, Sadovsky & Yaffe 1973), observer palpation (Hems 1973, Wood *et al* 1977), electromagnetic pressure sensors (Sadovsky & Yaffe 1973), strain-gauge devices (Wood *et al* 1977), tocodynometric transducers (Timor-Tritsch *et al* 1976) and piezo-electric crystals (Sadovsky *et al* 1977).

Ultrasound has been used to study fetal movement in the first trimester (Henner *et al* 1975, Reinold 1973, Jouppila 1976 and Kubli *et al* 1976) and A-scan ultrasound systems have been used to study fetal respiration (Boddy & Dawes 1975, Maršál & Gennser 1976). In the last few years real-time ultrasound has been used to study fetal respiratory movements (Maršál & Gennser 1976, Patrick 1977, Roberts *et al* 1977, Wladimiroff *et al* 1977, Manning 1977, Lewis 1977) and there have been some studies of fetal movement in the third trimester (Roberts *et al* 1977, Patrick 1977).

These studies have led to the belief that reduced levels of fetal movement and fetal respiration are indicative of fetal hypoxia, and that absent fetal movement or respiration is a sign of severe fetal distress that should be treated by immediate delivery of the fetus (Boddy & Dawes 1975, Sadovsky & Yaffe 1973, Pearson & Weaver 1976). One of the major problems in interpreting the data is that there is not enough information on the patterns of fetal activity in normal pregnancies in the third trimester.

For this reason we designed this study of normal pregnancies to investigate patterns of fetal body movement and fetal respiratory movement, the variations occurring in one fetus at different times of the day and the variations between different fetuses. As well as intensive 24-hour studies we have been collecting data from other normal pregnancies and more than 300 recordings in over 100 normal pregnancies.

We have also been studying patterns of fetal activity in growth-retarded fetuses and in the fetuses of mothers where the pregnancy is complicated by either severe hypertension or diabetes. We present data here from the first 20 growth-retarded fetuses that we studied. The diagnosis of growth retardation was made using ultrasound and later confirmed at delivery, and all studies of fetal activity were made using an ADR real-time scanner.

PATIENTS AND METHODS

The normal fetus

Twenty-one patients between 28 and 39 weeks gestation agreed to participate in the first study. All were normal in that there were no complications of pregnancy, they were non-smokers, took no drugs, were aged 18 to 32 years, and were all delivered of normal babies with no signs of fetal distress. All birthweights were between the 5th and 95th weight centile for gestational age (Thompson *et al* 1968).

Each woman was studied over a 24-hour period starting at 10.00 a.m. The 24 hours were split into 8 three-hour sessions during which FRM and FTM were observed for 45–60 minutes using a real-time scanner. The first ten patients were studied for two half-hour sessions with a 5-minute interval during which samples of blood were taken. The last eleven patients were observed continuously for a period lasting between 45 and 60 minutes. We felt that 60 minutes was the maximum period a woman could be expected to lie in the same position. During the remainder of the 24 hours the women were encouraged to go about their normal activities as much as possible. The patients slept on a bed in the scanning room so that there was little disturbance to mother and fetus when the transducer was placed in position. The light was switched off or dimmed during the night and most women slept during the evening scanning session. Meals were taken at regular hospital times; no special diet was arranged, and the patients were allowed to eat and drink as normal.

The transducer was placed on the mother's abdomen and a view obtained of a transverse section of the upper fetal abdomen. The women lay in a semi-recumbent position with a pillow under their right side to prevent them lying flat. All respiratory and body movements of the fetus were recorded. Respiratory movements were easy to identify and consisted of rhythmical movements of the fetal chest and abdomen. Hiccup-type movements were also recorded and were defined as sharp movements of the fetal chest and abdomen associated with a generalized jerking of the body occurring at a rate usually between 15 and 20 per minute in an irregular fashion. These movements were not recorded as breaths but were analysed separately by noting the times they started and finished in a separate log. Isolated limb movements with no movements of the fetal trunk were not recorded. It was our impression that most significant limb movements of the fetus were associated with movements of the fetal body. Thus there were some limb movements and some slight head movements that were not observed.

The transducer was held in place using a clamp designed and manufactured by Kretz-Technic UK. Each breath observed was punched directly onto computer tape using a hand-held punch, and the beginning and end of each fetal body movement was punched using a separate button. The tape was analysed by computer and calculations made of:

1 Fetal respiratory movements (FRM)
The fetus was defined as 'breathing' when the respiratory rate was 10 breaths per minute or more, i.e. a gap of greater than 6 seconds between breaths was defined as a cessation of respiration. The amount of time spent breathing was expressed as a percentage of the total observation time. The fetal respiratory rate was calculated from each two consecutive breaths by measuring the time interval between them. This was printed out for each observation period as a histogram of breath rates, but the results presented here are taken by evaluating the mean respiratory rate for each observation period.

Reproducibility studies of the ultrasound method were performed. Ten half-hour videotapes were analysed 'blind' by three separate observers and five half-hour videotapes were analysed three times by the same observer at intervals of greater than a week. With different observers the mean standard deviation in analysis of percentage FRM was 1.99%, and with the same observer it was 1.87%.

2 Fetal trunk movements (FTM)
As the beginning and end of each movement period was punched it was possible to measure the exact amount of time the fetus spent moving in any observation period, this was expressed as a percentage of the observation time. The total number of fetal movements observed was also recorded.

Reproducibility studies show that the mean standard deviation in analysis of percentage FTM was 1.98% with different observers and 1.25% with the same observer. The mean standard deviation of the number of moves was 5.03 moves in a 30-minute period with different observers and 3.04 moves with the same observer. The reproducibility for percentage FRM and percentage FTM was thus very good, but reproducibility for the number of moves was less good, the coefficient of variation being 18% with different observers and 9% with the same observer.

3 Total fetal activity (TFA)
Percentage incidence of TFA was defined as the amount of time the fetus spent either breathing or moving and was expressed as a percentage of the total observation time.

In the results section 'day' refers to 8.00 a.m. to 7.59 p.m., 'night' to 8.00 p.m. to 7.59 a.m. and 'post-prandial' to recordings made between 30 and 120 minutes after a meal.

PATIENTS AND METHODS

The growth-retarded fetus

Twenty patients with growth-retarded fetuses diagnosed by ultrasound were studied. In all the patients the abdominal circumference measurements were below the 5th centile limit for the stage of gestation, and all were at 28 weeks' gestation or more as confirmed by early ultrasound or certain dates. Three patients were defined as having symmetrical growth-retarded fetuses in that both head circumference and abdomen circumference were below the 5th centile limits with the head to abdomen circumference ratio within normal limits. Seventeen patients had asymmetrical growth-retarded fetuses in which the ratio of head circumference to abdomen circumference was abnormal (Campbell & Thoms 1977). At delivery all the babies were below the 5th centile in weight for their gestational age (Thompson *et al* 1968).

There were two still-births, one from a sudden abruptio, confirmed by a history of severe abdominal pain and evidence of a large retroplacental clot at the time of delivery. The other still-birth was due to intra-uterine hypoxia. Eighteen babies were born alive, fifteen by elective Caesarian section, one by Caesarian section following fetal distress in labour and two were normal vaginal deliveries. Fetal activity was studied using an ADR real-time scanner in the same manner as described earlier. In seven patients only one 40-minute recording was possible before delivery, in five patients intensive 24-hour studies were performed, and in eight patients serial recordings over periods ranging from several days to several weeks were possible. The minimum recording period was 40 minutes. The computer tape was analysed and calculations were made in a similar manner to that mentioned above. Six of the patients were smokers but they were asked not to have a cigarette for one hour before each recording period. Ten patients were on no drugs apart from haematinics. Seven patients had raised blood pressure and were either on hydrallazine, methyl dopa or both, one patient was diabetic on insulin, one patient was having heparin, one patient was on ritodrine/placebo trial, one was on a course of intramuscular dexamethazone and one patient for one recording had had amniocentesis the same day. One patient was on valium (*Roche*) 5 mg three times a day.

Antenatal cardiotocograph (CTG) recordings of 30 minutes' duration were made using an abdominal ultrasound transducer. These recordings were timed to occur within 24 hours of the recording of fetal activity and this was possible in 18 of the 20 patients. An abnormal CTG tracing was defined as one which showed late decelerations in response to Braxton Hicks' contractions associated with loss of beat to beat variation, absent fetal heart accelerations and little or no fetal movement as recorded by the mother. Ten abnormal CTG tracings in 6 patients were recorded. In all of those, except one, there were marked late decelerations in response to mild Braxton Hicks' contractions. In one patient there was a flat trace with no beat to beat variation, no fetal heart accelerations and no fetal movements recorded. All other tracings showed portions of good beat to beat variation, no decelerations and the mother recorded the presence of fetal movement during the recorded period. The absence of fetal heart acceleration in response to fetal movement was not accepted as a criterion of abnormality.

In seventeen of the 20 patients, 24-hour urinary oestriol collections were performed. Low levels were defined as any recording below the 5th centile limit for gestational age (Klopper & Diczfalusky 1969).

RESULTS: THE NORMAL FETUS

A total of 229 recordings of between 30 and 60 minutes' duration were made in 21 cases, an average of nearly 11 recordings per patient.

Fetal respiratory movement

FRM were present for a mean of 31% of the time with a range of 11–61% over 24 hours. The range for individual recording periods was 0–92%. There was a marked diurnal variation (Fig. 10.1), the incidence of FRM being least in the late evening and early morning and greatest in early evening. There was a statistically significant difference between the percentage incidence of FRM from 1.00 a.m. to 4.00 a.m., and 7.00 p.m. to 10.00 p.m. ($P < 0.001$); and also between 'day' and 'night' ($P < 0.001$). During the rest of the day there was an increased incidence of FRM 'post-prandially' ($P < 0.04$). There

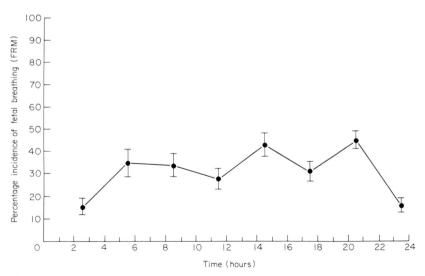

Fig. 10.1 The mean + standard error of the percentage incidence of fetal respiratory movements (FRM) in 21 normal pregnancies studied over a 24-hour period.

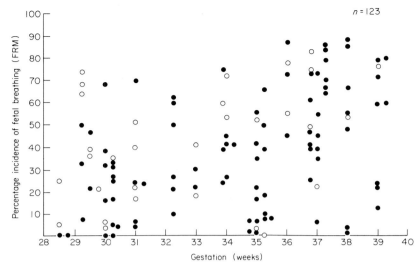

Fig. 10.2   All recordings of fetal respiratory movements (FRM) made during the 'day' (8.00 a.m.–7.59 p.m.) in 21 normal pregnancies plotted against gestational age. The open circles represent 'post-prandial' recordings (30–120 minutes after a meal)

was a wide variation at any particular hour of the day (Fig. 10.2) and it was not unusual to observe a normal fetus have periods of apnoea lasting 30 minutes. The mean percentage FRM in fetuses between 34 and 39 weeks was 34% and in those between 28 and 33 weeks was 27% ($P < 0.03$).

The mean respiratory rate was 43 breaths per minute (calculated only from the times in which breathing was taking place). The range for any particular time period was 16 to 133 breaths per minute. There was a significant difference between 'day' and 'night', with 44 breaths per minute during the 'day' and 40 breaths per minute at 'night' ($P < 0.008$). The mean 'post-prandial' breathing rate was 46 breaths per minute and this was not significantly different from the rate at other times of the day.

Fetal trunk movement

FTM were present for a mean of 18% of the time. This ranged from 11 to 26% over a 24-hour period, but for individual recordings ranged between 1% and 54%. There was a marked diurnal variation (Fig. 10.3), the incidence of FTM being greater in late evening and least around midday. There was a statistically significant difference between percentage FTM in the period 10.00 a.m. to 1.00 p.m. compared to the period 10.00 p.m. to 1.00 a.m. ($P < 0.001$), and also between 'day' and 'night' ($P < 0.001$). The incidence of FTM was less 'post-prandially' ($P < 0.007$).

Fetal trunk movements tended to be present in the absence of fetal respiratory movements and vice versa, though they did occasionally occur together. The mean incidence of concurrent respiratory movements and fetal

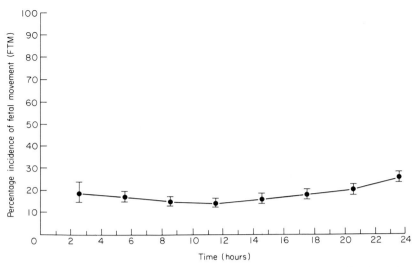

Fig. 10.3   The mean + standard error of the percentage incidence of fetal trunk movements (FTM) in 21 normal pregnancies studied over a 24-hour period.

trunk movements was 2%. The mean percentage FTM was the same throughout the third trimester.

The mean number of moves observed during a 30-minute observation period was 29 (range 3–108). Although the percentage FTM was the same throughout the third trimester, the total number of fetal moves was greater in those fetuses between 28 and 33 weeks gestational age. The mean number of moves in those aged between 34 and 39 weeks was 20 and in the former 41 ($P < 0.001$). This suggests that fetuses between 28 and 34 weeks have movements of shorter duration than those later in gestation.

Total fetal activity

The mean incidence of TFA was 48% and for any particular time period ranged from 5–96%. As can be seen in Fig. 10.4 it is rare for the percentage incidence of TFA to be below 10% in any one observation period during the 'day'. There was a diurnal variation, the incidence of TFA during the 'day' being 51% and during the 'night' 43% (Fig. 10.5). There was also a slightly increased incidence of fetal activity 'post-prandially' (53%), but this was not significant. The longest period of total inactivity observed was 17 minutes, the mean was 3 minutes with a standard deviation of 3.

Hiccups. Fetal hiccups were observed in seven patients. They lasted for periods of from 5 to 20 minutes and did not occur at any particular time of the day.

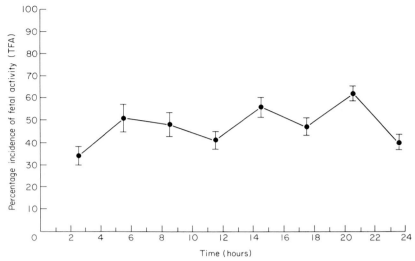

Fig. 10.4 The mean + standard error of percentage incidence of total fetal activity (TFA) in 21 normal pregnancies studied over a 24-hour period.

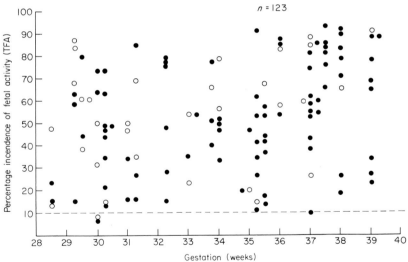

Fig. 10.5 All recordings of total fetal activity (TFA) made during the 'day' (8.00 a.m.–7.59 p.m.) in 21 normal pregnancies plotted against gestational age. The open circles represent 'post-prandial' recordings (30–120 minutes after a meal).

RESULTS: THE GROWTH-RETARDED FETUS

A total of 114 recordings were made in 20 patients. All recordings made on the same day have been grouped together and the results presented are a mean of these recordings.

Fetal respiratory movement

FRM were present for a mean of 16% of the time; this is significantly different from the mean incidence in normal fetuses ($P < 0.001$). In fourteen patients an incidence of less than 10% was recorded on at least one occasion (Fig. 10.6). This was associated with abnormal CTG tracings and low oestriols in three patients, with abnormal CTG tracings and normal oestriols in another three patients, with normal CTG tracings and low oestriols in one

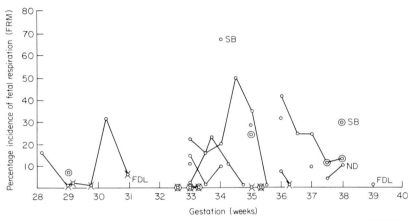

Fig. 10.6 The percentage incidence of fetal respiratory movements (FRM) in 20 growth-retarded fetuses plotted against gestational age. X represents abnormal cardiotocograph recordings; O low urinary oestriol levels; SB still-birth; FDL fetal distress in labour; ND normal delivery.

patient, and with normal CTG tracings and normal oestriols in the remaining six.

The mean respiratory rate was 41 breaths per minute which is not significantly different from the mean respiratory rate in normal pregnancies.

Fetal trunk movement

FTM were present for a mean of 12% of the time. This is significantly different from the incidence found in normal fetuses ($P < 0.001$). In seven patients a recording of FTM below 5% was made on at least one occasion (Fig. 10.7). In six of these patients there was an associated abnormal CTG trace and the seventh patient had fetal distress in labour as diagnosed by deep late fetal heart rate decelerations. Three of these patients had low oestriol recordings.

Total fetal activity

The mean TFA was 28%. This was significantly different from normal patients. Seven patients recorded an incidence of fetal activity below 10%

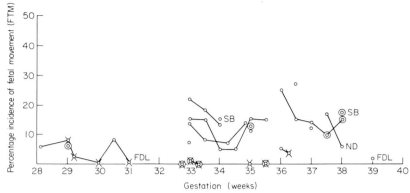

Fig. 10.7 The percentage incidence of fetal trunk movements (FTM) in 20 growth-retarded fetuses plotted against gestational age. X represents abnormal cardiotocograph recordings; O low urinary oestriol levels; SB still-birth; FDL fetal distress in labour; ND normal delivery.

(Fig. 10.8). In all of these there was an associated abnormal CTG trace and in one there was also fetal distress in labour as defined above. In three cases there were low oestriols. In all recordings above 10% fetal activity there were normal CTG traces but there were four patients with low oestriols. There were three fetuses with symmetrical growth retardation — their fetal activity was in the normal range.

There was no obvious correlation between drug ingestion or smoking and low fetal activity. Of the seven fetuses with TFA below 10%, two of the mothers were on hydrallazine, one on methyl dopa, one on insulin and dexa-

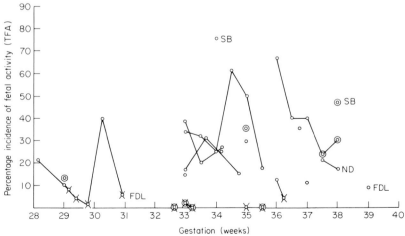

Fig. 10.8 The percentage incidence of total fetal activity (TFA) in 20 growth-retarded fetuses plotted against gestational age. X represents abnormal cardiotocograph recordings, O low urinary oestriol levels; SB still-birth; FDL fetal distress in labour; ND normal delivery.

methasone, and one on a placebo/ritodrine trial. Four were non-smokers and three smokers.

In two patients with a recording below 10% TFA, a drink containing 25 g of glucose was given but no significant change in fetal activity was noted.

CONCLUSION

A normal fetus appears to have patterns of alternating fetal respiratory movement, fetal body movement and total fetal inactivity. Fetal respiratory movements are greatest during the day and are much less in late evening and the early hours of the morning; the breathing rate is slightly greater during the day and after meals.

Fetal trunk movements are fairly constant during the day but increase in late evening. There is a significant increase in the latter part of the day and in the early hours of the morning. Different types of movement are observed but movements consist mainly of rotatory movements of the fetal trunk or sharp movements of the fetal body associated with kicking or punching movements. It is interesting to note that the fetuses in the gestation range 28–34 weeks seem to have shorter movement periods than those in the later gestation period. Fetal hiccups are very easy to distinguish from fetal respiratory movements and were observed in both normal and abnormal fetuses. The significance of fetal hiccups is as yet uncertain.

In considering whether fetal respiratory movements or fetal trunk movements may be of use as a clinical test of fetal well-being, it is important to notice the large range in incidence of both at any particular hour of the day. Analysing this data — even for recordings taken just during the day or postprandially — we still find that there are results which show a very low incidence of fetal respiration or a low incidence of fetal movement. The use of either of these variables as a single entity clinical test would almost certainly lead to a large number of false-positive recordings.

The recording for TFA, however, showed that it is rare for normal fetal activity to fall below 10% in any one half-hour period during the day and it is also rare for more than 10 minutes to elapse without any signs of fetal activity. Further studies in which we collected over 300 recordings from more than 100 normal patients confirm this early impression and it appears that it may be possible to define a lower limit of normal fetal activity at 10% and this may be useful as a clinical test.

In growth-retarded fetuses the percentage incidence of FRM, FTM and TFA is, in general, lower than in normal fetuses. There appears to be a good correlation between low levels of fetal activity and abnormal CTG traces. The correlation between oestriols and fetal activity was not good. Of the seven patients with TFA below 10%, five were delivered by elective Caesarian section, and two had fetal distress in labour as defined by deep late fetal heart rate decelerations in response to contractions. One was delivered by emergency Caesarian section and the other had a normal delivery despite the deep decelerations. In only two patients was the 5-minute Apgar score 7 or less. An umbilical artery pH was done at the time of delivery in only one case and was found to be 7.18. There was no fetal activity 2 hours prior to this Caesarian section.

More patients need to be studied to confirm the conclusion but it appears that a level of TFA below 10% correlates well with abnormal CTG recordings. This measurement of fetal activity is not subject to the variability of FRM or even FTM where low levels can be seen in normal fetuses and this may be a parameter that is useful in the detection of fetal distress and in the monitoring of the fetus which is at risk.

REFERENCES

BODDY K. & DAWES G. S. (1975). *Br. Med. Bull.* **31**, 3.
CAMPBELL S. & THOMS A. (1977). *Br. J. Obstet. Gynaecol.* **84**, 165.
HEMS D. A. (1973). *Bio Neonate* **23**, 223.
HENNER H. *et al* (1975). Proceedings of the 2nd European Congress of Ultrasonics in Medicine, Munich.
JOUPPILA P. (1976). *Acta Obstet. Gynaecol. Scand.* **55**, 131.
KLOPPER A. & DICZFALUSKY E. (1969) *Fetus and Placenta.* Blackwell Scientific Publications, Oxford.
KUBLI F., HALLER U. & HENNER H. (1976). *Lancet* i, 91.
LEWIS P. (1977). Fetal Breathing Meeting, Oxford.
MANNING F. A. (1977). *Postgraduate Medicine* **61** (4), 116.
MARŠÁL K. & GENNSER, G. (1976). Fetal Breathing Meeting, Oxford.
PATRICK J. (1977). Fetal Breathing Meeting, Oxford.
PEARSON J. F. & WEAVER J. B. (1976). *Br. med. J.* i, 1305.
REINOLD E. (1973). *J. Perinatal Med.* **1**, 65.
ROBERTS A. B., LITTLE D. & CAMPBELL S. (1977) Current Status of Fetal Heart Rate Monitoring and Ultrasound in Obstetrics, eds. R. W. Beard and S. Campbell. RCOG.
SADOVSKY E. & YAFFE H. (1973). *Obstet. Gynaecol.* **41**, 845.
SADOVSKY E. *et al.* (1977). *Int. J. Gynaecol. Obstet.* **15**, 20.
THOMPSON A. N., BILLEWICZ W. Z. & HYTTEN F. E. (1968). *J. Obstet. Gynaecol. Br. Commonw.* **75**, 903.
TIMOR-TRITSCH I., ZADOR I., HERTZ R. H. & ROSEN M. G. (1976). *Am. J. Obstet. Gynecol.* **126**, 70.
WOOD C., WALTERS W. A. W. & TRIGG P. (1977). *Br. J. Obstet. Gynaecol.* **84**, 561, 567.
WLADIMIROFF J. W., VAN WEERING H. K. & ROODENBURG E. (1977) The Current Status of Fetal Heart Rate Monitoring in Ultrasound and Obstetrics, eds. R. W. Beard and S. Campbell. RCOG.

CHAPTER 11

The future of real-time ultrasound in obstetrics

H. B. Meire

Recent progress in the development and clinical application of real-time ultrasound has been very rapid and most of the major advances could not have been forecast more than a year or two in advance. My task as real-time ultrasound prophet is thus very difficult and any major advances which may be revealed in the next year or so are unlikely to be accurately forecast in the following pages. Within the constraints of human fallibility however, a range of logical advances are foreseeable. Future developments can be divided into two types, technical and clinical. Even in the absence of further technical development there would be considerable room for improvement and extension of the clinical application of real-time scanning, but further technical progress should widen the clinical scope still further. I will therefore review the likely technical advances first and then discuss the possible extension of the clinical aspects of real-time.

TECHNICAL ADVANCES

Resolution

Current equipment is very much easier to use than the conventional, manually operated compound scanners but its major limitation to date has been inferior resolution. In order to consider how this is likely to be improved we must briefly review the different types of scanner that are available since the limitations and capabilities vary widely. Paradoxically the simpler (and hopefully less expensive) devices may well prove to have the best resolution. Scanners can be divided into sector scanners and linear scanners, the former viewing the tissue from a single point of contact and the latter over an extended length of contact. Sector scanners therefore view an arc of tissue whilst linear scanners view a rectangular volume. These two different types of equipment can be further subdivided into mechanical and electronic systems, though mechanical linear scanners are in a minority. The majority of linear scanners employ an array of multiple transducers which are fired off in sequence to produce the 'scanning' action. Sector scanners may also employ a small array of elements which are energized in a variety of complex sequences to steer the resultant ultrasound beam through an arc. Alternatively a single conventional type of transducer can be moved mechanically. We need not discuss the various types of mechanism which have been used for this to date though, in general, they consist of either an oscillating single transducer or a rotating wheel with multiple transducer crystals embedded in it. The wheel may have its moving surface exposed or be enclosed in an oil-filled capsule (see Fig. 1.28).

The resolution of all these systems depends essentially on the width of the interrogating ultrasound beam. It is a relatively straightforward matter to construct a single circular disc transducer with a long focal zone which is symmetrical about the transducer axis. These are the types of transducer currently used in conventional compound scanners. Conversely, the beam characteristics of the very small elements of the electronically controlled devices are much more difficult to predict, which makes control and symmetrical focussing almost impossible to achieve. This, therefore, is where the apparent paradox lies at the present. The simple, single element devices have better beam widths and therefore better resolution than the more complex and expensive multi-element scanners. Sophisticated electronic circuitry is already achieving considerable improvements in the focal characteristics of the multi-element devices and, by varying the delay between the firing of adjacent elements, it is possible to achieve focussing at selected depths during the transmission phase. Similar focussing can be employed in the reception mode also and, with still more complex circuitry, the 'focal zone' can be swept through the different tissue depths to improve focussing at a wide range of depths. Such apparatus is necessarily very expensive and the effective frame rate is reduced to about 5–10/sec. This may limit the acceptability of the image for the user. In addition, focussing is in a single plane only, and the lateral resolution resulting from the width of the array will remain unaltered. It is technically possible to improve this lateral resolution by using a mosaic of transducers in which complex delays between the energizing of different elements will permit the beam to be focussed at almost any depth and steered through a wide range of angles within a three-dimensional cone (dynamic focussing). The frame rate of such a device would be very slow indeed and its price proportionately higher.

In contrast to this electronic 'arms race' we have the single disc transducer. Whilst it is likely that further advances will be made in improving the beam profiles of these devices, a more dramatic improvement could be achieved by employing a transducer composed of concentric rings. By introducing an appropriate delay between the firing of each annulus, selective focussing can be achieved over a wide range of depths. The additional circuitry required and the manufacture of the transducer would increase the cost of this type of scanner, but it should still be less than that of the complex multi-element arrays and the resolution would be superior.

An additional factor which it is difficult to forecast is the improvement in design and manufacture of the controlling electronic circuits for multi-element arrays. Only recently has it been possible to produce relatively low cost variable delay devices and their size is rapidly being reduced. The use of purpose-built integrated circuits will reduce the size and cost of the electronic packages accompanying linear and phased arrays, but the likely balance between complexity and cost is very difficult to forecast. The more complex devices will almost certainly remain more expensive than the very satisfactory mechanical systems.

Image recording and memory

The human eye/brain combination integrates rapidly changing images into a smooth coherent moving image which has an apparent resolution that is better than that of each individual image. This is very evident when the otherwise acceptable 8 mm home movie images are viewed as stills, the grain size and lack of clarity are surprising. For the same reason the majority of users are disappointed in the quality of the still images obtained from real-time systems. A further disadvantage of many current scanners is the difficulty of obtaining images on any medium other than the rather expensive polaroid film.

The whole question of image recording is likely to become more important in the future. The main reason for this is related to the ease of use of real-time scanners. They will almost certainly be operated by technical or nursing staff who may have to diagnose possible abnormalities and probably also make a permanent record of other features such as the placental site. If necessary, the images can then be reviewed by the patient's obstetrician. The cost of polaroid would be prohibitive under these circumstances, but the available recording media costing perhaps one-tenth as much have slower photographic emulsions and require separate processing. The slower emulsions necessitate longer exposures and are thus unsatisfactory for recording live real-time images.

There are a number of possible solutions to these difficulties, the two most reasonable choices are using a digital memory and making the image compatible with a TV system. The latter can be achieved merely by placing a TV camera in front of the display screen, but there are two major disadvantages here: firstly, the smaller cameras have poor optical characteristics and introduce geometrical image distortion; secondly, the low brightness levels inherent in most display scopes necessitate a wide aperture in the camera optics with consequent loss of resolution and grey scale information. Low-light-level cameras are available but are generally more expensive than the more conventional ones.

A more satisfactory alternative is to perform the conversion to TV format electronically. This imposes constraints upon frame rate and line spacing with the linear scanners and cannot be applied directly to sector images. Some form of image memory then becomes necessary, and such a memory has besides many additional advantages (see below). Whilst conventional thermionic tube scan converters can be used as memories, they are bulky and have poor long-term stability. The use of a digital memory which can be smaller and should be free from long-term drift in its characteristics is a logical solution to this problem. The image can be written into the memory in whatever format or frame rate is desired and can be read out in conventional TV format. The further benefits of such a system are complete freedom from flicker, even at very slow frame rates, the ability to freeze the image at any time and the possibility of subjecting the image to electronic processing after it has been recorded. The ability to freeze an image is invaluable when one is seeking a particular structure such as the fetal spine or a limb. Photography can then be done at leisure and onto whatever recording medium is desired. A number of subsidiary advantages accrue from the use of the TV format including greater ease of demonstrating the image to an audience, especially for teaching purposes, and the ability to make good quality video tapes.

Digital memories capable of storing a single TV frame are just becoming available and it is therefore very likely that, in the near future, many real-time scanners will include these as a standard feature.

Size and cost

The question of cost has already been alluded to and financial trends are probably the most difficult to forecast. It seems likely, however, that continuing progress in electronic techniques will reduce the number of discrete components, despite increasing functional complexity. Manufacturing costs will therefore be held steady or reduced and the relative cost of the majority of real-time scanners will fall. In addition to these factors one must consider the current market trends. As clinical acceptance of real-time scanning increases, the potential market will expand and more manufacturers will join in. Competition normally pegs or reduces prices and increased production reduces manufacturing costs. I am therefore confident that a fairly wide range of real-time systems costing less than £10 000 will be available in the near future, some will cost only £5000 or possibly less. This is not to say that the more sophisticated electronic devices costing over £50 000 will cease to exist, but they will certainly find it increasingly difficult to justify their existence.

Concurrent with stabilization or reduction in price will be a reduction in the size of future systems. Many manufacturers have already incorporated the main transmitter electronics within the transducer housing and this trend will continue with inclusion of greater proportions of the electronic components until systems comprising a transducer assembly and display monitor only are the norm. One laboratory has already constructed a prototype unit in which the transducer lies at one end of a dumb-bell shaped, hand-held casing and the display monitor is mounted in the opposite end. The whole unit is self-contained and battery powered. The resolution is said to be very good and this unit may well herald the advent of the 'pocket' real-time scanner. Obviously there will be disadvantages in terms of image recording and viewing by more than one person, but such a system has many potential ergonomic advantages.

Hybrid scanners

At the opposite end of the scale one can see the development of sophisticated systems which may combine several different types of ultrasound techniques to solve particular clinical problems. Whilst basic imaging and fetal measurement are now fairly easily achieved, studies of fetal respiratory movements with real-time ultrasound require the presence of a dedicated, interactive operator if continuous records are to be obtained. Difficulties arise if there is fetal movement and I believe that the relative paucity of respiratory movements seen by some observers may suggest that low amplitude excursions are not detected. It is possible to construct a modification to a real-time scanner which will automatically follow the echoes from either side of the fetal chest and will accurately measure the distance between them. Such a system could be made to 'lock' onto predetermined echo complexes and to follow these during fetal movement. This would permit more or less continuous records of chest wall movement to be obtained with little, if any, operator interaction. In addition, it would permit the amplitude and velocity to be recorded instead of merely the frequency of movement.

A further possibility is incorporation of Doppler shift detection at predetermined loci within the field of view. This would permit a vessel to be located anatomically in real-time and its dimensions and the angle of its axis to the plane of transducer measured. Doppler measurements of the echoes from within the vessel would then permit blood velocity to be calculated and volume blood flow could then be computed. Applied to the fetal ductus venosus this would then permit quantitation of the fetal placental blood flow. It seems likely that this measurement would become abnormal in placental insufficiency.

There are doubtless many other special uses for which hybrid scanners could be designed and the future of this particular aspect of real-time scanning is indeed very exciting.

CLINICAL ADVANCES

The potential for the clinical exploitation of real-time ultrasound is only just being realized. Its development will rely partly on time and effort, even with current equipment, and partly on the further technical advances which I have mentioned above.

Experience to date suggests that the sector and linear scanners may have different clinical applications. These are determined by the shape of the field of view, the physical size and shape of the transducer assembly and the inherent image distortions produced by each system. In general, the sector scanners are preferable when one wishes to examine a small area in detail, whilst the linear arrays are better suited to reviewing a larger volume. Little has yet been written concerning the distortions inherent in real-time images but it is known that systematic geometrical aberrations are present (see Chapter 1). These are different for sector scanners and linear arrays and may invalidate measurements of fetal cross-sectional areas and circumferences.

With these factors in mind, I will now review the most likely areas for expansion of real-time imaging and suggest a few areas where its potential has not yet been tapped.

Routine antenatal scanning

For more than a decade a number of authorities have been emphasizing the potential value of routine ultrasound examination of all pregnant patients, preferably at the time of booking. This would permit early identification of multiple or grossly abnormal pregnancies and may permit identification of those patients who may subsequently have placenta praevia. The size and expense of conventional B-scanners has prevented them from being readily available in all units. This situation is aggravated both by the high degree of operator expertise necessary with this type of scanner and the relatively long examination time. The main advantages of real-time scanners are their ease and speed of operation. They are thus ideally suited for use in the antenatal clinic, particularly the smaller and less expensive versions. Interestingly enough, experience in my own department suggests that the more expensive electronic sector scanners are less suitable for use in obstetrics, whereas the linear arrays seem more satisfactory and cheaper. The main reason for this lies in the need to see the whole of the anterior uterine wall and this is obviously more easily achieved with a linear array. Balanced against this is the need to take some form of fetal measurement. It is certainly quicker and easier to obtain an accurate crown–rump length measurement with real-time, though the biparietal diameter may be less easy. If the fetal head is very low, posterior or steeply flexed it may be impossible to negotiate the fairly large linear array transducers into the correct position for visualization of the BPD. The smaller scanning head of the sector scanners is rather easier to position in these cases and may give a higher success rate. With this proviso, however, it seems reasonable to assume that the number of linear array scanners in use in antenatal clinics will (or should) increase rapidly in the near future. This may well result in an increase in referrals for conventional scanning if all cases with technically inadequate measurements or possible low placentae are referred.

The influence of real-time on the use of conventional machines for studying fetal growth is less easy to predict at the present. Certainly, adequate serial BPD measurements can be obtained with real-time, but modern ultra-sound practice is tending more towards measurement of trunk dimensions for the earlier detection of growth retardation. For these measurements to be useful the images have to be obtained at right angles to the fetal spine. This can be achieved with acceptable accuracy using a conventional scanner on which the plane of the fetal spine can be measured. With the freely mobile transducers used in real-time equipment there are no planes of reference and angles must be judged by eye. Compounding the sources of error here are the systematic image distortions mentioned above and the need to take the measurement from a polaroid print. This latter point is particularly relevant if no image magnification is available on the scanner. Measurement error increases enormously with smaller images. Whether or not these factors negate the value of trunk measurements by real-time scanners remains to be seen but I think it likely that, given adequate operator expertise, clinically useful measurements could be obtained. The availability of an image memory and magnification facility would improve the accuracy of the measurement, but these features are unlikely to be present on the type of scanner used in antenatal clinics.

Fetal abnormalities

The majority of abnormalities occur sporadically, though those patients with a family history or previous abnormal child may be at higher risk. The search for fetal abnormality, especially neural tube defects, should therefore ideally be aimed at the whole obstetric population. The sheer magnitude of this undertaking again indicates the need for a rapid examination, i.e. a real-time scan. The resolution of the early commercially available real-time scanners was not adequate to visualize the fetal spine in sufficient detail during the first trimester of pregnancy. Whilst it is possible to detect gross defects such as anencephaly, a functionally severe lumbar spina bifida may be overlooked.

From the viewpoint of patient management it is preferable to try to estab-lish an early diagnosis so that termination may be offered; real-time scanning is not yet capable of achieving this. However, as the resolution of systems improves, our ability to identify smaller defects must also improve and rou-tine first trimester screening for neural tube defects will soon become a reality.

The majority of other congenital abnormalities are less common than neural tube defects (in the UK), occur sporadically and exhibit less gross morphological defects. Population screening, by ultrasound at least, is there-fore not practicable at the present nor in the near future.

Modern genetic counselling departments, however, attract a high propor-tion of patients with a previous history of an abnormal child and ultrasound will have an increasing role to play in the management of these patients. Again, one is limited to those cases where a fairly gross morphological anom-aly is likely. Experience in this field is limited as yet, but a high-frequency, high-resolution real-time ultrasound scanner has been used in our department to inspect the fetal ventricular septum in a patient with a previous child with Ellis–van Creveld Syndrome. The fetal limb bones can also be seen and measured. As equipment and expertise improve, the scope and application of this form of imaging will widen, though the balance between the use of real-time and conventional scanners is difficult to predict.

CONCLUSION

The future prospects of real-time ultrasound seem bright. The ease and speed with which diagnostically adequate images can be acquired will ensure this. There are, nevertheless, a wide range of further technical developments which will improve the performance and thus the clinical value of these devices. The acceptance of real-time scanning as a regular part of the antenatal booking clinic routine is already technically feasible. The only major barriers are finance, staffing and the need for more concrete information confirming the clinical value of this concept. There is also, as yet, insufficient experience upon which we can base an assessment of the accuracy of real-time for the diagnosis of fetal abnormalities. However, those of us who have gained some experience with the existing equipment are fairly certain that reliable diagnosis of gross anomalies is almost within our grasp.

The continuing technical developments will not be conducted in the absence of development of other types of scanner. The performance of manually-operated compound scanners has improved remarkably in recent years and will doubtless continue to do so. I am therefore not of the opinion that real-time ultrasound will completely eclipse or supplant conventional scanning. Both will have a place in the obstetrics of the future, the conventional devices being used where high resolution or lack of geometrical distortion are of paramount importance.

As a radiologist, I must point out that the advent of real-time scanning is also expanding the non-obstetric uses of ultrasound, though here especially the conventional scanner will always have a role to play.

Index